The
ALCHEMY
of
YOU

Health secrets of phenomenal women.

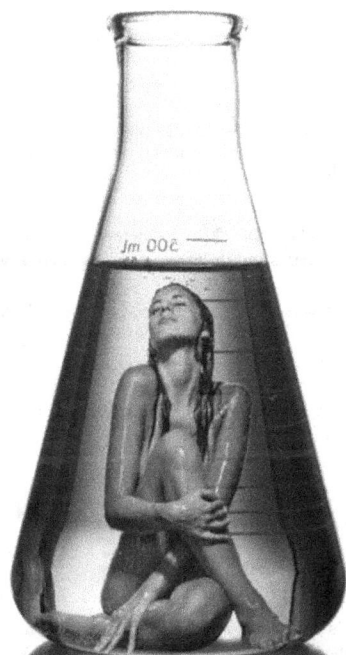

Patricia Copley O'Connell

NOVEL INSTINCTS

NOVEL INSTINCTS PUBLISHING
6008 Ross Avenue
Dallas, Texas 75206
www.novelinstincts.com

www.HormoneGuru.com

ISBN: 978-0-9726007-6-7

Cataloging information: 1. Women's Health 2. Menopause 3. Aging 4. Longevity
Library of Congress Control Number: 2011925818

Printed in the United States of America.
10 9 8 7 6 5 4 3 2 1

IMPORTANT NOTICE – PLEASE READ

The information in this book is for educational and entertainment purposes only and is NOT a substitute for qualified medical or professional evaluation, guidance or treatment. The author and publisher specifically disclaim any and all liability related to the use of this book.

Every effort has been made to ensure the accuracy of the information contained herein; however, no claims are made by the author or publisher regarding either the book's completeness or its accuracy. Readers are urged to conduct their own relevant research and to consult appropriate professionals before taking any health-related actions. The reader agrees that she/he is solely responsible for any actions she/he may take as a result of reading this book or any potion thereof.

*T*o all the women who thought they had lost themselves.

Welcome back!

TABLE OF CONTENTS

Acknowledgements

The author would like to thank the many people who have contributed to the development and improvement of this book. Particular thanks go to the various focus group members who described candidly what they wanted and needed in a resource like this. They are: Jeannie Brady, Cheryl Carter, Danee' Diaz, Carly Dunson, Kathy Harris. Mikka James, Angela Jiura, Ashley Linnabery-Sotello, Molly McCreary, Caren Mitchell, Tisha Muntz, Nancy Nevil, Cheryl Rivera, Laurie Roberts, Laura Simmons, Donna Starford, Laurie Stoekert, Vickey Wade, Beth Wood, Shannon Worthy and Blanche Stephens. I owe much gratitude to my brilliant designer, Paul Black, and the team at Novel Instincts publishing for their unerring class and professionalism. Smooches to my agents, Cricket Freeman and Jeffery McGraw of The August Agency, for their ongoing advice, perspective and delightful friendship though the years. Many thanks to Dr. Kelly Martin and Dr. Jill Wade for spurring me to write this long-overdue follow-up to my first book and for their tireless efforts to deliver smarter health solutions to their patients. My writer's group also deserves a special mention for their brainstorming and business advice and for raising the bar for us all. And there is no way to adequately show my appreciation to my vast circle of family and friends for your support and encouragement, so I just offer my continued love and give thanks for the blessings you bring me. Here's to my grown-up baby girl, Megan, her daughter Jordan, my many sisters, nieces, and all the young women who I hope will have better choices in part because of what this book has done.

INTRODUCTION

8O

What You Need to Know to Get the Results You Want

Alchemy is the fabled ancient art of using mystical substances to perform seemingly impossible tasks—like turning lead into gold or extending longevity.

Today we know this ancient practice by a more familiar name: *science*. Yes, modern science can now transform one element into another, and it can also tell us how to live longer, healthier lives.

But for most of us, this knowledge has remained hidden behind layers of myth and misdirection promoted by certain drug companies that want us to believe we have no power over our present and future wellbeing.

Well I'm here to tell you they are wrong. Like Dorothy in Oz, you've had the power all along and now's the time to take back control.

The Alchemy of YOU shows you how your internal chemistry affects nearly every aspect of your mind and body. And it tells you how to naturally manipulate that chemistry and the systems that drive it to maintain your health, vibrancy and youthfulness for a delightfully long time.

Yes, the secrets to staying young and feeling good are right here at your fingertips, all in one place, ready and waiting for you.

Audience

The Alchemy of YOU was created specifically for women of any age, especially those over 35, who are experiencing unwelcome changes in their overall health, including one or more common issues such as:

- Brain fog, memory loss
- Weight gain, difficulty losing weight, carb/sugar cravings
- Menstruation problems (irregular, long, heavy), severe PMS
- Insomnia, poor quality sleep
- Hot flashes, night sweats, racing heart, itchy skin
- Loss of (or dramatic surge in) sex drive and other passions
- Signs of aging in skin, hair, nails
- Indigestion, heartburn, acid reflux
- Fatigue, weakness

Objectives

The three most important things you should know right from the beginning are:

- You are not alone.
- You may not have to accept those changes.
- There are healthy and natural ways available to help prevent or reverse many dysfunctions we used to think were inevitable signs of aging.

The objective of this book is to empower and enable you to take a stronger role in your own wellness and to help shape the nature of your care.

Using the tools presented here, you will be able to:

- Identify and understand the tests that can help focus your quest for answers.

- Identify root causes for many of your symptoms.

- Rule out suspected causes based on test results and other symptoms.

- Identify a range of solutions — including human-friendly, natural solutions — that may reverse or minimize your most troublesome problems.

- Evaluate solutions to determine which are most compatible with your attitudes and life goals.

- Discuss with your doctor or healthcare advisor the directions you'd like to take in further exploring causes and solutions.

- Make grounded, knowledgeable decisions regarding your body.

How to Use This Book

This book is for informational purposes only. I encourage you to conduct your own research to learn more about the subjects presented here. And please be sure to consult a physician or other healthcare advisor for guidance in selecting and implementing any health-related solution.

Designed as a quick reference, *The Alchemy of YOU* is structured to make it as easy as possible for you to quickly find out what you can do about the issues you're currently dealing with and how to keep your body and mind in prime condition for the long run.

READ, LEARN, PLAN FOR ACTION

Read it once all the way through so you know how your systems and organs work together to keep your body purring like a well-tuned Ferrari. Then refer back to specific sections as you need them.

Or skip directly to the parts you need and read the rest later.

MAKE NOTES

I encourage you to mangle this book. Make notes in the blank areas, highlight or underline key points in the text, circle important sections, dog-ear pages, use paperclips or sticky notes to mark chapters and specific pages you want to refer back to, even photocopy certain pages to take to your doctors.

This is your book. Do whatever it takes to make it work for you.

TAKE AN ACTIVE ROLE

If you are happy following whatever healthcare advice you have been getting so far, then you don't really need this book.

On the other hand, if you would like to become a more active partner in charting your own healthcare course, then use the tools offered here to help you effectively — and respectfully — collaborate with your doctors and other healthcare advisors.

Organization and Content

I don't expect you to run out and implement every solution in the book. In fact, that would be both reckless and costly.

I trust that you will approach your issues thoughtfully, seeking to implement only the solutions that seem to offer the widest range of benefits that matter to you — the "biggest bang for the buck" — and that make the most sense to your healthcare advisors.

The structure of *The Alchemy of YOU* helps you do just that.

Following this *Introduction* chapter, the book is divided into four main parts (A-D), each with its own supporting chapters.

- **PART A (Problems).** Search the handy tables in the first part of the book to find specific problems that are bothering you — whether they are symptoms you've experienced or diagnoses you've been given based on previous tests or examinations. Identify any tests that may help point you toward specific causes. And search the list of possible solutions that might work for you.

- **PART B (Tests)**. Learn more about the types of tests available to help you focus in on the cause(s) of your concern.

- **PART C (Health Processes)**. Discover the four key processes/systems that interact to keep you healthy and youthful. And learn about the organs and glands that support or drive those processes. This knowledge will help you understand the causes of dysfunction and aging and how to prevent or reverse them.

- **PART D (Solutions)**. Here you will find detailed information about each of the most beneficial solutions. This will help you identify the top few solutions that can address the greatest number of your most troublesome issues.

Common Myths and Misconceptions

Knowledge about wellness and longevity is advancing at a staggering rate today. It's no wonder so many of us are confused.

The following will test your knowledge on some of the most common myths and misconceptions. These statements are typical of the advice or warnings you may get from the media, your friends, and other sources.

Mark the desired column to indicate whether you think each statement of advice or warning is valid (YES) or not valid (NO). (*Answers follow.*)

Common Myths and Misconceptions

YES	NO	TYPICAL ADVICE / WARNING
		You shouldn't take estrogen because it causes cancer.
		Estrogen increases your risk of stroke.
		If you take hormones, you should take the lowest dose for the shortest amount of time.
		If you don't have hot flashes you don't need to take hormones.
		Sunlight causes skin cancer.
		Cholesterol is bad for you.
		You need drugs like Fosamax or Boniva to prevent or treat osteoporosis.
		You can't be menopausal if you're still getting periods.
		Estrogen is the only hormone women need at menopause.
		People who supplement testosterone to youthful levels are like drug addicts getting high on hormones.
		Menopausal hormone therapy is dangerous.
		It's normal to feel sick, tired, weak, stupid, fat and sexless at your age.

ANSWERS

You shouldn't take estrogen because it causes cancer.

✗ False (with caveats)

Although your doctor may have other valid reasons not to prescribe estrogen for you, you should know that natural human estrogen *that is properly balanced by progesterone* typically *does not cause* cancer. (We'll discuss *horse* estrogens and *fake* progesterone later.)

In the normal process of growth and repair, your body occasionally makes mistakes, like typos in an email, and it randomly produces cells with mutated DNA. Your immune system routinely attacks any random mutants and makes those cells commit suicide (apoptosis).

If you're exposed to certain carcinogenic agents (like radiation or toxic substances), they may damage the DNA of a large number of exposed cells and thus increase the odds that any given cell division will produce a mutant cell.

Imagine your immune system is like a server at a restaurant. It can keep up with the normal number of customers when the normal number of staff are on duty. But if several servers are out sick, even with a normal crowd, it will be hard for the few servers on duty to keep up. And if the customer volume doubles or triples unexpectedly, even when all the usual staff are on duty, you can be sure that some of those customers will end up neglected and angry.

Like that unusually large crowd of diners, sometimes so many mutant cells are generated at once (by radiation, toxins, drugs, etc.) that your healthy immune system can't keep up.

And if your immune system is compromised by stress, too little sleep, poor nutrition, or illness, it may not be able to keep ahead of the even the normal number of mutants.

For the immune system, either scenario can lead to cancer, and the odds are even greater when both scenarios occur at the same time.

Highly simplified, cancer is a collection of mutated cells that have bonded together to support the cluster/tumor's spread, and to form defenses against your immune system.

Because estrogen is designed to stimulate cell division and growth (of eggs in the ovaries, of the uterine lining, of milk glands in the breasts) it increases the number of randomly occurring mutants, simply because it promotes more rapid cell division. But it *does not necessarily cause the mutations.*

The progesterone your body makes when you ovulate each month calms estrogen's tendency to stimulate cell growth. When estrogen is "opposed" by high enough quantities of progesterone each month, the progesterone protects you from developing estrogen-sensitive cancers by simply limiting the rate of cell division to keep it within a range your immune system was designed to handle.

Think of it this way: If estrogen caused cancer, then women who have been pregnant should be at the highest risk for hormone-related cancers. Right?

But just the opposite is true: pregnancy actually *reduces* the lifetime risk of hormone-related cancers. Perhaps that's because although the most important strong estrogen (E2/estradiol) increases dramatically during pregnancy, it is balanced by a *two times greater* increase in progesterone.

Estrogen increases the risk of blood clots.

✓ True

Estrogen *alone* does promote clotting, and higher estrogen levels do indeed increase the risk of blood clots. In fact, pregnant women may be at an increased risk of getting blood clots if their estrogen levels are not properly balanced by progesterone.

Progesterone normalizes the clotting process. (During pregnancy, progesterone rises by 300 times normal, versus estrogen's 100-times increase.) So it's very important to have just the right balance of estrogen and progesterone.

If you take hormones, you should take the lowest dose for the shortest amount of time.

✗✓ Not necessarily

In the wake of the Women's Health Initiative (WHI) — which studied the effects of *horse estrogen* (Premarin) and *horse estrogen plus fake progesterone* (Prempro) in menopausal women — the FDA issued a requirement to include warnings on *all* pharmaceutical hormone products (including bio-identical hormones, which are chemically identical to those our bodies naturally make).

And they cautioned doctors to prescribe those products to women in the "lowest effective dose for the shortest amount of time." But what's "effective" can differ dramatically from one woman to the next.

Furthermore, this action did not take into consideration studies that show the benefits and safety of using bio-identical hormone replacement therapy (HRT).

Neither did it acknowledge the fact that it may actually be the (largely *reversible*) hormone *imbalances and deficiencies* — which occur naturally as we get older—that predispose us to a variety of what are falsely assumed to be "age-related" conditions.

We now know that restoring hormones to optimal levels can help *prevent* many of the conditions and diseases typically blamed on aging and can keep you looking and feeling youthful.

If you don't have hot flashes there's no reason to take hormones.

✕ False

Many women brush off discussions of hormone supplementation as irrelevant to them because they don't have hot flashes.

All women should understand that as we age our hormones drop off at different rates, causing imbalances whose damaging effects may not become apparent for decades or may not be properly attributed to hormone dysfunction.

For example, a breast cancer tumor (triggered by estrogen that is not balanced by enough progesterone) can take 7-10 years to grow large enough to detect.

Although the tumor may not be discovered until after a woman enters menopause, it may have been "born" when she was in her 40s and was having irregular cycles. Those crazy periods were a signal that she was not ovulating every month, and that her body was not making enough progesterone to balance her estrogen.

The lack of symptoms creates a false sense of security. We need to be aware of our hormone imbalances early and correct them to prevent the diseases that may crop up later.

Symptoms that many women assume are inevitable and unrelated—such as insomnia, fatigue, weight gain, loss of muscle/skin tone, depression, even heart disease, cancer, arthritis and osteoporosis—may in fact be preventable or reversible by restoring their hormones to optimal levels.

Sunshine causes skin cancer.

✓✗ Not necessarily

You would think that people who live in sunny tropical climates should have the highest incidence of skin cancer, but you would be wrong.

In fact, deadly melanoma (along with other cancers) is far more prevalent among those who live closer to the poles and have *less* exposure to sunlight.

Your body was designed to produce vitamin D in your skin when exposed to UV rays and sweat. Depending on the color of your skin (dark skin blocks more UV rays than light skin), you can produce between 10,000 and 20,000 IUs of vitamin D3 on a sunny summer day...assuming you expose enough skin and don't cover it with sunscreen.

Study after study shows that vitamin D3 is critical to the fight against a whole host of cancers as well as heart disease, autoimmune diseases, osteoporosis and others.

But what have you heard for years regarding sunshine? *"Stay out of the sun.* And if you have to be out there, *cover up and wear sunscreen."* The current recommended amount of vitamin D3 is 800 IUs, which is woefully inadequate, considering that you were designed to run on 10,000 to 20,000 a day. If you are avoiding all sunlight on your skin, then you will have to get the vitamin D you need from somewhere else.

Some of us think that if we drink milk and consume other products fortified with vitamin D we are getting enough. But not all sources provide the right kind of vitamin D, and those that do don't provide enough. The vitamin we need to be our healthiest is D3, and we need a lot of it.

Fortunately, even mainstream experts are now beginning to acknowledge the benefits of vitamin D3 and are recommending we get at least 1000-2000 IUs per day. Some doctors even supplement vitamin D3 in single doses upwards of 60,000 IUs to quickly restore patients who are severely deficient.

Even TV's Dr. Oz has recommended getting about 10 minutes a day of direct sunlight on unprotected skin. That's a breakthrough in thinking. Following his recommendation could dramatically reduce the occurrence of a variety of deadly diseases over the next few decades, especially for today's young people.

But keep in mind that as you age, your skin becomes much less effective at producing vitamin D even under optimal conditions. By the age of 70 you may be producing only 25% of the amount you made when you were younger. So vitamin D supplementation becomes even more important with each year.

Cholesterol is bad for you.

✗ False

We all know the cholesterol story is complex and there are good and bad types of cholesterol.

What you may not know is that *cholesterol is essential to the normal function of your body*. It is the raw material from which many of your hormones are made. If it is too low, you cannot make the hormones that keep you alive. It is so important, in fact, that most of your cholesterol is made in your liver. Only a portion of the cholesterol in your blood comes from your diet.

Cholesterol alone is not bad for you, but *oxidized* cholesterol is—which is why it is important for you to get plenty of *anti*oxidants like vitamin C, resveratrol, curcumin, and others.

Even the American Heart Association admits that total cholesterol is a poor indicator of cardiovascular health. What is most important (and you'll notice this is a theme running throughout this book) is that you *maintain the proper balance* of cholesterol levels, ideally through exercise and diet.

As it turns out, inflammation is far more damaging to your heart. And indicators of inflammation like homocysteine and

C-reactive protein (CRP) may tell you more about the condition of your cardiovascular system than cholesterol levels.

Keep in mind that the statin drugs typically prescribed for high cholesterol are well known to damage the liver and deplete the body of an essential nutrient, CoQ10.

And—according to a recent meta-analysis of 11 studies, published in the *Archives of Internal Medicine* (June 28, 2010)— although statins may be effective in lowering cholesterol levels and reducing the number of myocardial infarctions, *they have not been shown to reduce the overall risk of dying!*

Drugs provide the best treatment for osteoporosis.

✗ False

Healthy bone constantly undergoes a process of breaking down and rebuilding. Your hormone levels and their ratios to one another are critical to keeping this remodeling process in perfect balance.

Estrogen is responsible for slowing the rate of bone loss, while progesterone, testosterone and growth hormone are responsible for building new bone.

Osteoporosis drugs tend to work like estrogen to preserve existing bone. But they don't provide the other components that help build strong, resilient new bone.

In fact, the best way to maintain strong bones is a 4-pronged approach:

1. Consume the building blocks of bone (calcium, magnesium, vitamin D3, protein, etc.)

2. Maintain optimal hormone levels needed for bone remodeling (estrogen, progesterone, testosterone, and perhaps growth hormone).

3. Keep body pH slightly to the alkaline side of neutral.

4. Get regular weight-bearing exercise.

If you must take bone-preserving medications, you must also continue to support your bones in other ways.

You can't be menopausal if you're still getting periods.

✓× Technically true, but misleading

Traditionally, menopause has been defined as the point at which a woman has had no natural periods for 12 consecutive months.

While accurate, this definition fails to acknowledge the condition of *hormonal* menopause, when a woman's FSH (produced in the brain) is continuously above 25 mIU/mL and her estradiol (the most important form of natural estrogen) falls below 50 pg/mL.

A woman who is hormonally menopausal may continue to have periods—though they are likely to be irregular, sometimes very heavy or long lasting—while suffering symptoms like hot flashes, insomnia, brain fog, and others typical of classical menopause.

Estrogen is the only hormone women may need at menopause.

× False

Women and men are both built to run on the same hormones, including estrogen, progesterone and testosterone. But women typically have a lot more estrogen than men, and men have a lot (10 times) more testosterone than women. And for both sexes, it is critical to maintain the proper balance of hormones.

For example, because estrogen is also produced in fat cells (as well as the ovaries and adrenal glands), a heavy post-menopausal woman may not need to take estrogen. But she *will* need progesterone to balance the estrogen her body still makes. She may also need testosterone to boost her brain, build muscle and bone, or bring back her passions.

Although every woman is different, the one hormone almost all women need in the years leading up to and following menopause is *progesterone,* because we have no significant backup sources for progesterone after our ovaries shut down or are surgically removed.

People who supplement testosterone to youthful levels are like drug addicts getting high on hormones.

✗ False

No one would accuse a diabetic of "getting high" on his insulin, or would call someone a "thyroid addict" because she supplements hormones for her underactive thyroid.

And yet, when it comes to supplementing sex hormones, it happens every day.

A recent news story featured a doctor from a world-renowned hospital insisting that people, like our local police chief, who replenish their depleted testosterone supplies are equivalent to narcotic addicts.

The ignored fact is that testosterone is an essential hormone for brain function, bone and muscle integrity, heart health, assertiveness, and sex drive.

Testosterone deficiency has been linked to the development of Alzheimer's and Parkinson's diseases. In other words, supplementing testosterone to bring it back up to optimal levels may actually *prevent* these terrible diseases.

Do people with low testosterone feel a kind of "high" when they finally begin to restore their hormone levels? Sure. If someone has tried to suffocate you, do you feel a kind of "high" when you catch that first breath upon release? Absolutely. Does that make you an *air addict*? No.

It's true that athletes and others may abuse this hormone. But when used properly, it can be a blessing...for men *and* women.

Menopausal hormone therapy is dangerous.

✓✗ May be true in some circumstances, but not all

Whenever someone tells you that studies have proven hormone replacement therapy (HRT) is dangerous, there is one very important question you need to ask: "What specific hormones are you talking about?"

What few people realize is that *virtually all the large studies of HRT over the past 70 years have focused primarily (or exclusively) on the use of hormones that are foreign to the human body!*

Whether a given study intentionally examined only specific HRT hormone products, or merely tracked the use of HRT among large groups of women, the fact is that, *until the early 2000s, nearly all women on* HRT were using Premarin (if they had no uterus) or Prempro (if they still had a uterus and needed a form of progesterone to balance the strong estrogens in Premarin).

And as we've discussed earlier, Premarin is made from horse estrogen, while Prempro is Premarin plus the synthetic progesterone substitute called Provera (or MPA).

So, when someone says, "All the studies show that estrogen [or progesterone]..." does certain things (good or bad), they typically mean that *horse estrogen* or *fake progesterone* has been shown to do those things.

The fact is that NONE of the major HRT studies often cited reflect the impact of either our *human hormones* or the *bio-identical versions* of those hormones that are made from plants and are *chemically identical* to human hormones.

However, at least one large study (2005 French E3N study of 54,000 women) now helps to balance this picture, showing significant benefits and reduced risks associated with the use of bio-identical hormones.

It's normal to feel bad at your age.

✓✗ It may be true but it doesn't have to be

Too often we are judged by what's normal "for our age." Some will say it's normal to be slowing down or to have a few health complaints at a certain age. Our blood tests may come back saying that our hormone levels are "perfectly normal"...*for someone in the age bracket where hormones are typically low!*

It's a crazy kind of circular logic that fails to address the difference between "normal" (meaning what typically occurs in the average population) and "optimal" (meaning *ideal*).

Maybe it's a holdover from the time when doctors couldn't do anything about the inevitable changes that come with age. But we've advanced since then and have the tools to restore our bodies in many ways to their optimal conditions.

In the past, we thought of aging as synonymous with a decline in health. But in fact they are two separate things.

Yes, certain things occur as a function of age. But a great many of the complaints that bother us as we get older are the result of hormone imbalances and other circumstances that we can prevent or counteract.

The Top 2 Health Secrets for Women

Now that you've had a taste of some of the royal secrets, you can see that there is a lot more to learn. In the pages of this book, you'll find many great solutions, some that apply to most women, and others that apply to only a few.

But there are two supplementation solutions *every woman should know about, especially as she gets older*:

- Bio-identical progesterone
- Vitamin D3

Both progesterone and vitamin D are *hormones* (really!) manufactured in your body when the conditions are right.

- Progesterone is made (from cholesterol) in the ovaries (and in the placenta during pregnancy).

- Vitamin D is made in the skin when exposed to the sun's UV rays and sweat.

Unfortunately, the mechanisms that produce each of these hormones don't always work reliably, especially as we age. And sometimes we disable them by our well-intentioned actions. So here's what you can do to get back on track.

KEY BENEFITS OF THE TOP 2 SECRETS

Both of these substances will be described in greater detail in Part D. Here's just a glimpse into their extraordinary benefits:

PROGESTERONE BENEFITS

- Prevent estrogen-sensitive cancers
- Prevent/reduce PMS
- Calm irregular/heavy periods
- Increase metabolism
- Promote weight loss
- Decrease appetite
- Normalize clotting
- Ease anxiety/depression
- Build strong bones, muscles
- Improve brain & memory
- Support heart/cardio health
- Promote sleep
- Support sex drive
- Reduce allergies

VITAMIN D3 BENEFITS

- Prevent most cancers
- Protect against melanoma
- Manage diabetes
- Improve bowel function
- Minimize chronic pain
- Tame MS, rh arthritis, etc.
- Improve immune system
- Build strong bones, muscle
- Promote heart health, lower BP
- Prevent stroke
- Support brain/memory
- Promote healing, slow aging
- Support eye health
- Reduce gum disease

You can see why these two solutions deserve special emphasis.

PROGESTERONE SNAPSHOT

- If you are not ovulating regularly, or if your ovaries have been removed, *your body cannot produce enough progesterone to balance the estrogen it continues to make in your adrenal glands and fat cells.*

- If you test low in progesterone relative to estrogen (especially in what should be the second half of your menstrual month, or after menopause), you should supplement progesterone to prevent "estrogen-dominance" cancers and many degenerative conditions.

- You can get natural creams over the counter (in health food stores, online, etc.) that contain pharmaceutical-grade, bio-identical (same as what nature gave you) progesterone.

VITAMIN D3 SNAPSHOT

- *Melanoma (skin cancer) rates are **higher** among those who get the **least sun**,* whether because of their location (nearer the poles the sun's UV rays are weaker), or because they wear cover-ups and sunscreen.

- Our bodies manufacture the vitamin D hormone in our skin when it is exposed to UV rays and sweat. But with age, our skin loses much of that ability, making only about 25% as much vitamin D from sunlight by the time we reach our 70s.

- Depending on our skin color, we can produce as much as *10,000 to 20,000 IUs of vitamin D just by being out in the sun—* with plenty of skin exposed and no sunscreen on a summer day in warmer latitudes. Just 15 minutes a day may give us all the vitamin D we need.

- Because burns and overexposure to the sun can *also* cause certain skin cancers and exaggerate the appearance of aging, more and more doctors are recommending that most people who avoid the sun take at least 1000-2000 IUs of vitamin D3 a day to stay healthy.

- Vitamin-D-fortified milk and foods may contain D2, which is the wrong kind of vitamin D. (Always look for vitamin D3.)
- Optimal vitamin D3 levels—as measured by the 25(OH)D blood test—should be around 60-80 ng/mL.

...And So the Quest Begins

You've seen how facts can be misinterpreted and have already discovered a few of the key secrets of human chemistry that phenomenal women possess.

Now you are ready to embark on the quest to find your own best solutions to keep you healthy, youthful and vibrant for years to come.

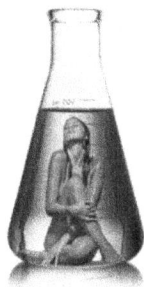

PART A: **PROBLEMS**

2| Problems Desperately Seeking Solutions

You have needs. This book has solutions. PART A of *The Alchemy of YOU* gets you from one to the other in a flash, without a lot of fuss.

Quick-Reference Format

Each chapter in this first section addresses a group of related issues that may concern you. These are presented in a three-column table format for easy reference.

- The **left column** lists the symptoms, **problems**, conditions and diagnoses that may concern you.

- The **middle column** indicates common **causes** for those issues.

- And the **right column** lists a variety of actions or **solutions** you might implement.

This book does not cover conventional solutions the doctors on your team are likely to suggest. It assumes those bases are covered. Neither does it delve into exotic or rare causes for various symptoms.

Instead, it focuses on the many *common* causes that may either be overlooked or simply disregarded as untreatable or unworthy of treatment. And it suggests the complementary solutions that may be appropriate for those conditions.

The solutions entries often begin with a list of tests, each designed to help you home in on the true cause of the problems.

Then they suggest a range of preventive or corrective solutions that may apply to your issues.

Later in the book you will learn more about tests and possible solutions as well as the overall systems/processes and organs that keep your body operating at its best.

Symptoms Everyone Should Recognize

Before getting into your specific issues, let's take a moment to talk about four potentially deadly conditions (heart attack, stroke, ovarian cancer and endometrial cancer) whose symptoms may be overlooked.

In some cases these are clusters of otherwise very mundane symptoms that can be attributed to simpler causes. Sometimes it is only as a group that these ordinary symptoms reveal something more sinister.

HEART ATTACK

We all know the classic signs of a heart attack in men: shooting pain in the left arm, a crushing feeling in the chest and shortness of breath.

But we women don't like to do things the way men do. A woman having a heart attack is much more likely to be misdiagnosed than a man because her symptoms often look like other, less serious, conditions.

So here are the symptoms to watch for:
- Pain in left arm/chest, jaw, back or stomach
- Sudden unexplained anxiety/fear
- Shortness of breath
- Sudden heavy sweating/cold sweat,
- Lightheadedness, sleep disturbances
- Indigestion, nausea

- Severe fatigue, muscle aches

STROKE

Many people can avoid the damaging effects of a stroke if they carry aspirin with them and take one or two tablets at the first indication of trouble.

When someone is having a stroke it is important to get the right kind of help (including aspirin) administered within the first 45 minutes. After that, they are more likely to suffer permanent damage.

Symptoms of a stroke can include:
- Crooked smile or facial asymmetry, one side drooping
- Slurred speech
- Weakness, numbness or loss of control on one side
- Difficulty walking
- Lost or diminished vision
- Sudden, severe headache
- Sudden confusion

To respond when you think someone is having a stroke, think of the word FAST.

- *Face*: Ask for a smile.

- *Arms*: Ask them to hold both arms out straight.

- *Speech:* Ask them to repeat a familiar phrase

- *Time*: Act fast! Have them take aspirin as soon as possible, then call 911 or get them to an ER ideally within 15 minutes.

OVARIAN CANCER

Like pancreatic cancer, ovarian cancer is so deadly because it reveals no obvious symptoms early on and cannot be found in routine screenings.

So it is important to watch for these ordinary symptoms that, together as a group, may be subtle signals of ovarian cancer:

- Abdominal bloating and/or pain
- Pelvic pain
- Fatigue
- Indigestion
- Urinary frequency
- Constipation

Some people believe the CA-125 test is a good way to find ovarian cancer early. It isn't. As a screening tool, it produces a lot of false alarms and misses about half of actual cancers.

Unfortunately, it is primarily useful only in confirming a late-stage diagnosis of cancer and in tracking the effectiveness of cancer treatment, according to experts at Johns Hopkins University and elsewhere.

Currently, the best way to screen for ovarian cancer may be through ultrasound examinations, though this is certainly not a foolproof test.

Some women may even choose to have their ovaries removed once they shut down at menopause in order to prevent this insidious disease.

ENDOMETRIAL CANCER

The number-one symptom of cancer of the uterine lining (endometrial cancer) is *irregular bleeding*.

And *any bleeding after natural menopause is considered a sign of endometrial cancer* until proven otherwise.

However, if you are peri- or post-menopausal with an intact uterus and are taking supplemental hormones, you could continue having periods indefinitely. In that case, the diagnosis of cancer becomes much more difficult.

To watch for this deadly disease after menopause, get regular pelvic exams that include transvaginal ultrasound and possibly biopsy.

It's All About You Now

You've learned about the structure of this chapter and have gathered some handy tips for spotting symptoms of four of the most deadly conditions.

Now, it's time to think about what's bothering you.

Identifying your specific symptoms, issues and conditions is the first step on the path toward finding the answers (and secrets) you've been looking for.

YOUR CONCERNS

Use this page to list your problems, issues, concerns, conditions
and diagnoses that need solutions.

_____

_____

_____

_____

_____

_____

_____

_____

_____

_____

_____

_____

_____

_____

_____

_____

_____

_____

_____

_____

3| Allergies & Immune Dysfunctions

PROBLEM	COMMON CAUSES	POSSIBLE SOLUTIONS
IMMUNE DYSFUNCTION **new or worsening allergies, asthma, hives, autoimmune conditions**	▪ Food sensitivity /leaky gut syndrome ▪ Parasites or yeast/Candida ▪ Low progesterone ▪ Hormone allergies ▪ Adrenal fatigue/ stress ▪ Drug reaction	*Conduct tests* ▪ Food allergies ▪ Elimination diet ▪ Hormone allergy ▪ Progesterone ▪ Adrenal function *Address the cause(s)* ▪ Cleansing ▪ Rotation diet ▪ HCL, probiotics, enzymes ▪ Add progesterone ▪ High-dose vitamin C, zinc, curcumin ▪ Hormone desensitization ▪ Allergy shots ▪ Alternative drug ▪ Reduce stress *Address the symptoms* ▪ Antihistamines ▪ Corticosteroids ▪ Malic acid

Allergies and Immune Dysfunctions (cont.)

PROBLEM	COMMON CAUSES	POSSIBLE SOLUTIONS
FREQUENT COLDS, INFECTIONS	• Weakened or compromised immune system • Stress/adrenal fatigue	*Address the cause(s)* • Vitamin D3, C, zinc, quercetin • Other immune-boosting supplements • Reduce stress • Improve sleep
COLD SORES, fever blisters, shingles	• Herpes virus • Weakened or compromised immune system • Stress/adrenal fatigue	*Address the cause(s)* • Vitamin D3 • Vitamin C, quercetin • Immune-boosting supplements • Reduce stress • Improve sleep *Address the symptoms* • Lysine, arginine • Lip treatments • Calamine lotion • Antihistamines

4| Appearance: Skin, Hair

PROBLEM	COMMON CAUSES	POSSIBLE SOLUTIONS
AGING SKIN, dry, thinning, sagging skin, loss of elasticity	• Low/imbalanced sex hormones • Low/imbalanced thyroid hormones • Low growth hormone (GH) • Sun damage	*Conduct tests* • Sex hormones • Thyroid hormones • GH/IGF-1 • Allergy blood test *Address the cause(s)* • Add/balance sex/ thyroid hormones • Quercetin, B-complex, resveratrol *Address the symptoms* • Reduce sun exposure • Lotions, oils
AGE SPOTS, scaly skin,	• Low/imbalanced sex hormones • Low/imbalanced thyroid hormones • Poor nutrition • Normal end of cell life • Low growth hormone (GH)	*Conduct tests* • Hormones: sex, thyroid, GH (IGF-1) • Micronutrients *Address the cause(s)* • Add and/or balance sex/thyroid/growth hormones • Multivitamin, esp. vitamin C, D3, E, zinc • Resveratrol, calorie restriction diet *Address the symptoms* • Reduce sun exposure • Lotions • Laser treatment

Appearance: Skin, Hair (cont.)

PROBLEM	COMMON CAUSES	POSSIBLE SOLUTIONS
HAIR LOSS, thinning hair, receding hairline	• High/imbalanced testosterone (plus hereditary male pattern baldness) • Thyroid imbalance • Low stomach acid	*Conduct tests* • Testosterone • Thyroid *Address the cause(s)* • Add/balance sex/thyroid hormones • Reduce testosterone • Add HCL *Address the symptoms* • Hair growth products • Follicular transplant
COARSE, GRAY HAIR	• Normal aging (i.e., low catalase enzyme, excess systemic hydrogen peroxide) • Thyroid imbalance • B12 deficiency • Smoking	*Conduct tests* • Thyroid • B12 *Address the cause(s)* • Balance thyroid • B12 (and folate) • Quit smoking • *[Watch for new tests & products addressing catalase enzyme and peroxide]* *Address the symptoms* • Hair dyes, conditioners
THICK SKIN	• Low thyroid	*Conduct tests* • Thyroid hormones *Address the cause(s)* • Balance thyroid

Appearance: Skin, Hair (cont.)

PROBLEM	COMMON CAUSES	POSSIBLE SOLUTIONS
EXCESS FACIAL & BODY HAIR	▪ High/imbalanced testosterone ▪ Thyroid imbalance	*Conduct tests* ▪ Testosterone ▪ Thyroid *Address the cause(s)* ▪ Balance hormones ▪ Reduce testosterone *Address the symptoms* ▪ Waxing, shaving, electrolysis
MISSING EYEBROWS	▪ Thyroid imbalance	*Conduct tests* ▪ Thyroid hormones *Address the cause(s)* ▪ Balance thyroid *Address the symptoms* ▪ Cosmetics ▪ Tattooing
ACNE	▪ Excess or imbalanced testosterone (*see Ovarian Cysts/PCOS*) ▪ Yeast/Candida	*Conduct tests* ▪ Testosterone ▪ Yeast *Address the cause(s)* ▪ Balance/reduce testosterone ▪ Cleansing *Address the symptoms* ▪ Tetracycline, etc. ▪ Acne products ▪ Skin cleansing

Appearance: Skin, Hair (cont.)

PROBLEM	COMMON CAUSES	POSSIBLE SOLUTIONS
BRITTLE, PEELING NAILS	▪ Nutritional deficiency ▪ Hypoxia (smoking) ▪ Allergy to fish scales used in some glittery nail polish	*Conduct tests* ▪ Micronutrients *Address the cause(s)* ▪ Nutritional therapy, esp. vitamin C, calcium *Address the symptoms* ▪ Nail strengthener ▪ Avoid glittery nail polish
SKIN TAGS	▪ Excess dietary sugar/carbs ▪ Insulin resistance (possibly type 2 diabetes) ▪ Adrenal fatigue ▪ Estrogen dominance	*Conduct tests* ▪ Blood sugar ▪ Cortisol ▪ Sex hormones *Address the cause(s)* ▪ Diabetic diet ▪ Adrenal therapy ▪ Balance sex hormones *Address the symptoms* ▪ Surgical removal
RED NECK (often with white area in center)	▪ Cause currently unknown; common in menopausal women	*Address the symptoms* ▪ Makeup ▪ Laser treatment

5 | Brain & Mood

PROBLEM	COMMON CAUSES	POSSIBLE SOLUTIONS
BRAIN FOG, poor memory, difficulty concentrating	• Low/imbalanced sex hormones • Thyroid dysfunction/ imbalance • High cortisol • Low cortisol (adrenal burnout/ "pregnenolone steal") • Low growth hormone (GH) • Nutritional deficiencies • Drug side effect (esp. statins, CoQ10 depletion)	*Conduct tests* • Sex hormones • GH/IGF-1 • Thyroid hormones • Adrenal function *Address the cause(s)* • Add/balance sex hormones, &/or GH • Thyroid therapy • Adrenal therapy • Add pregnenolone • Brain-support supplements • Reduce stress • Add/lower cortisol • Low-dose lithium • Avoid statins or add CoQ10 *Address the symptoms* • Brain exercise • Memory tricks & techniques

Brain & Mood (cont.)

PROBLEM	COMMON CAUSES	POSSIBLE SOLUTIONS
DEPRESSION, no/low enthusiasm, low passions, low ambition, senses dull	• Sex hormone imbalance • Low testosterone • Insufficient exercise • Nutritional deficiencies • Seasonal affective disorder (SAD) • Neurotransmitter imbalances in brain	*Conduct tests* • Sex hormones • Micronutrients *Address the cause(s)* • Balance hormones • Add testosterone • Exercise • Nutritional therapy • Light therapy • Mood-stabilizing supplements
IRRITABILITY, mood swings	• Sex hormone imbalance • High testosterone • Thyroid dysfunction • Low growth hormone (GH)	*Conduct tests* • Sex hormones • GH/IGF-1 • Thyroid hormones *Address the cause(s)* • Add/balance sex hormones • Thyroid therapy • Add GH *Address the symptoms* • St. John's Wort, SAMe

Brain & Mood (cont.)

PROBLEM	COMMON CAUSES	POSSIBLE SOLUTIONS
ANXIETY, generalized feelings of fear/dread	• Fear-inducing life circumstances • Sex hormone imbalance • Toxicities • Nutritional deficiencies	*Conduct tests* • Sex hormones • Toxins • Micronutrients *Address the cause(s)* • Resolve fearful circumstances • Add/balance hormones • Cleanse/detox, chelation *Address the symptoms* • Cruciferous vegetables (broccoli, cauliflower, cabbage, Brussels sprouts, etc.) • Counseling
MUSIC STUCK IN YOUR HEAD (broken record syndrome, "ear worms," auditory memory loops)	• Unknown; may be related to hormones including stress hormones cortisol and/or adrenalin	*Conduct tests* • Sex hormones • Cortisol • Neurological *Address the cause(s)* • Add/balance hormones • Reduce stress • Take cortisol reducing supplements such as Relora, phosphatidyl serine *Address the symptoms* • Avoid music

6 | Discomfort & Pain

PROBLEM	COMMON CAUSES	POSSIBLE SOLUTIONS
HOT FLASHES, night sweats, clammy skin, heart racing (palpitations), electric shock sensation	▪ Low estrogen or estrogen withdrawal	*Conduct tests* ▪ Sex hormones (especially estradiol and progesterone) *Address the cause(s)* ▪ Add estrogen *Address the symptoms* ▪ Black cohosh ▪ Adaptive behaviors ▪ Exercise ▪ Weight loss
ITCHY, CRAWLY SKIN, feeling like you have bugs on your skin or scalp	▪ Low estrogen or estrogen withdrawal	*Conduct tests* ▪ Sex hormones *Address the cause(s)* ▪ Add estrogen ▪ Balance hormones
COLD ALL THE TIME, low body temperature	▪ Low thyroid hormones ▪ Adrenal dysfunction	*Conduct tests* ▪ Thyroid hormones ▪ Adrenal function *Address the cause(s)* ▪ Add thyroid hormone(s) ▪ Adrenal therapy

Discomfort and Pain (cont.)

PROBLEM	COMMON CAUSES	POSSIBLE SOLUTIONS
HEADACHES, migraines	• Sex hormone imbalance • Food triggers • Magnesium/B12 deficiency • Temporomandib-ular joint disorder (TMJD), grinding teeth, etc.	*Conduct tests* • Sex hormones • Elimination diet • Micronutrients *Address the cause(s)* • Add/balance sex hormones • Chiropractic therapy • Rotation/elimination diet • Magnesium, B-12 • 5-HTP, feverfew • *See Jaw Popping, Ch 8.*
MUSCLE CRAMPS, foot/leg cramps	• Low or high potassium • Other electrolyte imbalance • Sex hormone imbalance/ high testosterone • Diuretics or heart medications • Muscle strain	*Conduct tests* • Metabolic panel blood tests • Sex hormones *Address the cause(s)* • Add/balance potassium or other electrolytes • Alternative meds • Add/balance sex hormones • Stretch before exercise *Address the symptoms* • Massage, walk
VAGINAL DRYNESS, painful intercourse	*See Chapter 7: Menstrual & Sexual.*	

Discomfort & Pain (cont.)

PROBLEM	COMMON CAUSES	POSSIBLE SOLUTIONS
DRY EYES *(For dry mouth, see Chapter 8)*	▪ Sex hormone imbalance ▪ Sjogren's disease ▪ Side effect of drugs	*Conduct tests* ▪ Sex hormones *Address the cause(s)* ▪ Add/balance sex hormones ▪ Alternate drugs *Address the symptoms* ▪ Eye drops, ointments ▪ Punctal plugs
DIZZINESS, lightheaded-ness, vertigo	▪ Adrenal fatigue ▪ Inner ear infection or dysfunction ▪ Allergies ▪ Low aldosterone hormone	*Conduct tests* ▪ Adrenal function ▪ Allergies (blood/skin) ▪ Aldosterone *Address the cause(s)* ▪ Adrenal therapy ▪ Allergy therapy ▪ B-complex ▪ Add aldosterone *Address the symptoms* ▪ Ginger (for nausea) ▪ Guaifenesin ▪ Chiropractic therapy ▪ Low-dose Valium ▪ Ginkgo biloba, lesser periwinkle
BLOATING, swelling, water retention	▪ Low progesterone ▪ Food allergies/ sensitivities	*Conduct tests* ▪ Sex hormones ▪ Food allergies *Address the cause(s)* ▪ Add progesterone ▪ Elimination diet

Discomfort & Pain (cont.)

PROBLEM	COMMON CAUSES	POSSIBLE SOLUTIONS
BLADDER INFECTIONS, urinary tract infections (UTIs)	▪ Bacterial contamination *(from intercourse, toilet, tight pants, etc.)* ▪ Estrogen dominance	*Address the cause(s)* ▪ Genital/sexual hygiene ▪ Balance sex hormones ▪ Antibiotics *Address the symptoms* ▪ D-mannose ▪ Cranberry ▪ Azo/pyridium
BODY/JOINT ACHES, pain in shoulders, neck or low back	▪ Spinal dysfunction ▪ Autoimmune disease, inflammation, arthritis ▪ Damaged joints ▪ Bacterial infection ▪ Food allergies/sensitivities ▪ Nutritional deficiencies ▪ CoQ10 depletion (from statins) ▪ Adrenal fatigue	*Conduct tests* ▪ X-rays ▪ Chiropractic ▪ Rheumatology exam ▪ Orthopedic exam ▪ Bacterial labs ▪ Micronutrients ▪ Food allergies ▪ Adrenal *Address the cause(s)* ▪ Chiropractic therapy ▪ Reduce inflammation ▪ Vitamin D3 ▪ Nutritional therapy ▪ Rotation diet ▪ Avoid statins or add CoQ10 ▪ Adrenal therapy *Address the symptoms* ▪ Glucosamine, chondroitin, MSM ▪ High-dose omega-3 oils

Discomfort & Pain (cont.)

PROBLEM	COMMON CAUSES	POSSIBLE SOLUTIONS
LEAKING URINE, incontinence	• Loss of urinary muscle tone • Low/imbalanced sex hormones • Bladder nerve spasms • Bladder/ureter weakness	*Conduct tests* • Sex hormones • Urology exam *Address the cause(s)* • Add/balance sex hormones • Drugs to quiet spasms • Bladder suspension surgery *Address the symptoms* • Incontinence pads • Pelvic floor and bladder-retraining exercises
TINGLING EXTREMETIES, numbness in hands, feet	• Poor circulation • Diabetic neuropathy • Drug side effect (esp. from chemotherapy or statins) • Carpal tunnel syndrome (possibly B6 deficiency) • Spinal misalignment, nerve impingement • Nutritional deficiency • Stress	*Conduct tests* • Circulation • Nerve conduction • Micronutrients • Chiropractic *Address the cause(s)* • Diabetes treatment • Alternative drugs • Chiropractic therapy • Glutamine • Nutritional therapy: B complex, esp. B6 (pyridoxamine) • Add CoQ10 • Reduce stress

Discomfort & Pain (cont.)

PROBLEM	COMMON CAUSES	POSSIBLE SOLUTIONS
RINGING IN EARS (tinnitus)	• Underactive thyroid • Allergies • Sex hormone imbalance • Drug side effect • High blood pressure • Oral infection • Zinc deficiency	*Conduct tests* • Thyroid hormones • Allergies • Sex hormones • Hearing • Blood pressure *Address the cause(s)* • Add thyroid hormones • Add/balance sex hormones • Allergy shots • Alternative drugs (or supplements) • Reduce blood pressure • Dental/periodontal treatment • Add zinc *Address the symptoms* • Ginkgo biloba, black cohosh • Stress-reducing techniques, meditation • Hypnotherapy

7| Menstrual & Sexual

PROBLEM	COMMON CAUSES	POSSIBLE SOLUTIONS
CRAMPS, severe PMS	• Calcium &/or magnesium deficiency • Low progesterone (from failure to ovulate) • Hormone allergy	*Conduct tests* • Sex hormones • Hormone allergy *Address the cause(s)* • Calcium and/or magnesium supplements • Add progesterone • Hormone desensitization *Address the symptoms* • Anti-inflammatory, painkiller drugs
IRREGULAR CYCLES, clotting/heavy periods, long periods	• Low progesterone (from failure to ovulate)	*Conduct tests* • Progesterone *Address the cause(s)* • Add progesterone

Menstrual & Sexual (cont.)

PROBLEM	COMMON CAUSES	POSSIBLE SOLUTIONS
SKIPPED PERIODS	• Low body weight, low body fat • Excessive exercise, overtraining • Failure to ovulate, and/or sex hormone imbalance • PREGNANCY	*Conduct tests* • Sex hormones • Pregnancy *Address the cause(s)* • Add/balance sex hormones • Gain weight • Moderate training
INFERTILITY, miscarriage	• Low progesterone • Sex hormone imbalance *(or lack of coordination between estrogen and progesterone cycles)* • Reproductive structural anomalies	*Conduct tests* • Sex hormones • Ob/gyn exam *Address the cause(s)* • Add progesterone • Surgical intervention • Fertility solutions
YEAST INFECTIONS	• High estrogen and/or testosterone • Genital environment (underwear traps moisture) • Body pH (acid/alkaline) imbalance • High sugar/simple carbs diet • Antibiotic use	*Conduct tests* • Sex hormones • Yeast • pH (urine or saliva) *Address the cause(s)* • Reduce testosterone • Balance pH • Genital hygiene • Breathable panties, loose pants • Vaginal medications • Diabetic diet • Avoid antibiotics *Address the symptoms* • Vaginal creams

Menstrual & Sexual (cont.)

PROBLEM	COMMON CAUSES	POSSIBLE SOLUTIONS
REDUCED NIPPLE SENSITIVITY	• Low testosterone, imbalanced sex hormones	*Conduct tests* • Sex hormones *Address the cause(s)* • Add/balance sex hormones • DHEA supplements
SORE, SENSITIVE NIPPLES	• Sex hormone imbalance • Temporary effect of newly restored hormones	*Conduct tests* • Sex hormones *Address the cause(s)* • Add/balance sex hormones
SAGGING BREASTS	• Sex hormone imbalance • Low growth hormone (GH)	*Conduct tests* • Sex hormones • GH/IGF-1 *Address the cause(s)* • Add/balance sex hormones • Add growth hormone
FIBROCYSTIC BREASTS	Specific causes unknown. Contributors can include: • Excess caffeine • Low progesterone	*Conduct tests* • Mammogram, sonogram • Sex hormones • Iodine *Address the cause(s)* • Eliminate caffeine • Iodine

Menstrual & Sexual (cont.)

PROBLEM	COMMON CAUSES	POSSIBLE SOLUTIONS
LOSS OF SEX DRIVE (libido), diminished sexual fantasy/desire, reduced ability to orgasm	▪ Low testosterone ▪ Sex hormone imbalance ▪ Sexual trauma	*Conduct tests* ▪ Sex hormones *Address the cause(s)* ▪ Add testosterone ▪ Add/balance sex hormones ▪ DHEA ▪ Counseling, sex therapy
VAGINAL DRYNESS, painful intercourse	▪ Low estrogen ▪ Low testosterone	*Conduct tests* ▪ Sex hormones (especially estradiol and testosterone) *Address the cause(s)* ▪ Add estradiol (vaginal or systemic) ▪ Add testosterone *Address the symptoms* ▪ Vaginal lubricants
BLADDER INFECTIONS (UTIs)	*See Chapter 6: Discomfort and Pain.*	

8| Mouth, Eyes, Nose, Ears

PROBLEM	COMMON CAUSES	POSSIBLE SOLUTIONS
BLEEDING GUMS, red, inflamed gums (gingivitis)	• Periodontal disease • Low vitamin C, zinc • Vitamin C withdrawal • Adrenal fatigue	*Conduct tests* • Periodontal exam • Micronutrients • Adrenal function *Address the cause(s)* • Periodontal treatment • Vitamin C, zinc • Adrenal therapy
CAVITIES, tooth decay	• Poor dental hygiene • Excess sugar in diet • Decreased saliva • pH imbalance	*Conduct tests* • Dental exam • pH dipstick *Address the cause(s)* • Brushing/flossing • Diabetic diet • pH balancing *Address the symptoms* • Dental treatment
HEART DISEASE	• Inflammation from chronic/untreated periodontal disease	*See Chapter 12: Conditions and Diagnoses.* *See Bleeding Gums, above.*

Mouth, Eyes, Nose, Ears (cont.)

PROBLEM	COMMON CAUSES	POSSIBLE SOLUTIONS
BURNING TONGUE/ MOUTH	• Decreased saliva *(see Dry Mouth)* • Low/imbalanced sex hormones • Nutritional deficiency • Nerve dysfunction	*Conduct tests* • Sex hormones • Micronutrients • Nerve conduction *Address the cause(s)* • Add/balance sex hormones • Nutritional therapy • Chiropractic therapy *Address the symptoms* • Tooth/mouth numbing products
BAD BREATH, bad taste in mouth	• Nutritional deficiencies • Iron-deficiency anemia • Bleeding gums • Bacterial overgrowth • Extreme weight loss/ketosis	*Conduct tests* • Micronutrients • Blood count • Periodontal exam *Address the cause(s)* • Nutritional therapy • Iron supplements • Periodontal treatment *Address the symptoms* • Tongue scraping • Mouthwash
DRY MOUTH, too little saliva	• Sex hormone imbalance • Drug side effect	*Conduct tests* • Sex hormones *Address the cause(s)* • Add/balance sex hormones • Alternate drugs *Address the symptoms* • OTC mouth moistening products

Mouth, Eyes, Nose, Ears (cont.)

PROBLEM	COMMON CAUSES	POSSIBLE SOLUTIONS
INCREASED/ DECREASED SENSE OF SMELL	• High/low testosterone • Certain drugs • Cold, sinus infection • Migraines • Nerve dysfunction, spinal misalignment	*Conduct tests* • Testosterone • Nerve conduction • Chiropractic exam *Address the cause(s)* • Add/reduce testosterone • Alternate drugs or supplements • Migraine treatment • Chiropractic therapy
JAW PAIN / POPPING	• Temporo-mandibular joint disorder (TMJD) • Allergies/ inflammation • Jaw misalignment	*Conduct tests* • Dental exam, x-rays • Allergies *Address the cause(s)* • Allergy desensitization • Anti-inflammatory supplements • Dental splint • Chiropractic therapy • Therapeutic massage • Acupuncture • Botox injection in jaw

Mouth, Eyes, Nose, Ears (cont.)

PROBLEM	COMMON CAUSES	POSSIBLE SOLUTIONS
MACULAR DEGENER-ATION (eyes)	• Excess antacid use • Low stomach acid • Nutritional deficiency • Low/imbalanced sex hormones • Excitotoxins (like MSG, aspartame, etc.)	*Conduct tests* • Micronutrients • Sex hormones *Address the cause(s)* • Added HCL • Avoid antacids • Nutritional therapy, esp. selenium, zinc, lutein • Add/balance sex hormones • Detox
HEARING LOSS	• Adrenal fatigue • Low aldosterone • Nerve impingement	*Conduct tests* • Adrenal function • Aldosterone *Address the cause(s)* • Adrenal therapy • Chiropractic therapy • Aldosterone hormone
RINGING IN EARS (tinnitus)	*See Ch 6: Discomfort & Pain.*	
MUSIC STUCK IN YOUR HEAD	*See Ch 5: Brain and Mood.*	

9 | Sleep, Strength & Energy

PROBLEM	COMMON CAUSES	POSSIBLE SOLUTIONS
INSOMNIA, poor quality sleep	• Low/irregular estrogen levels • Stress/excitement (excess adrenalin or cortisol) • Low melatonin • Excess light in bedroom • Overactive thyroid	*Conduct tests* • Sex hormones • Thyroid hormones • Adrenal function/ cortisol *Address the cause(s)* • Add/stabilize estradiol • Improve sleep hygiene • Melatonin • Exercise gently before bed • Reduce stress • Iodine *Address the symptoms* • Add progesterone • Cortisol-lowering supplements • Valerian
DIZZINESS UPON STANDING	• Adrenal fatigue	*Conduct tests* • Adrenal function *Address the cause(s)* • Adrenal therapy

Sleep, Strength &Energy (cont.)

PROBLEM	COMMON CAUSES	POSSIBLE SOLUTIONS
MUSCLE WEAKNESS, difficulty building muscle	• Estrogen dominance, low testosterone, and/or low progesterone) • Low DHEA • Overactive thyroid or goiter • Adrenal fatigue • Low growth hormone (GH) • Nutritional deficiencies	*Conduct tests* • Sex hormones & DHEA • Thyroid function • Adrenal function • GH/IGF-1 • Micronutrients *Address the cause(s)* • Add testosterone, progesterone, DHEA • Thyroid treatment • Adrenal therapy • Add GH • Nutritional therapy
TIREDNESS, fatigue, low energy, exhaustion	• Adrenal fatigue, adrenal burnout • Low/imbalanced sex hormones • Low B vitamins • Nutritional deficiencies • Low/imbalanced thyroid hormones • Heavy metal/ other toxicity • Low growth hormone (GH)	*Conduct tests* • Adrenal function/ cortisol, DHEA • Sex hormones • Thyroid hormones • Micronutrients • Toxicity/hair analysis • GH/IGF-1 *Address the cause(s)* • Reduce stress • Adrenal therapy • B vitamins (esp. B12 & folate/folic acid) • Improve sleep • Add/balance sex/ thyroid hormones • Cleanse/chelation

10 | Weight & Digestion

PROBLEM	COMMON CAUSES	POSSIBLE SOLUTIONS
WEIGHT GAIN, excessive hunger, carb/sugar cravings	• Low/high/ imbalanced sex hormones • Low thyroid • High cortisol, adrenal fatigue • Insufficient exercise • Nutritional deficiencies • Poor diet	*Conduct tests* • Sex hormones • Thyroid hormones • Adrenal function • Micronutrients *Address the cause(s)* • Add/balance sex/ thyroid hormones • Adrenal therapy • Reduce cortisol • Nutritional therapy/diabetic diet • Reduce stress • Exercise • DHEA • Chromium • Iodine
DIABETES	*See Chapter 12: Conditions & Diagnoses*	
EXCESSIVE WEIGHT LOSS	• Overactive thyroid, goiter • Adrenal fatigue	*Conduct tests* • Thyroid function • Adrenal function *Address the cause(s)* • Iodine • Thyroid treatment

Weight & Digestion (cont.)

PROBLEM	COMMON CAUSES	POSSIBLE SOLUTIONS
FOOD INTOLERANCE, alcohol intolerance	• Food sensitivities • Adrenal fatigue • Low stomach acid (HCL) • Low digestive enzymes	*Conduct tests* • Elimination diet • Adrenal function • Food sensitivies *Address the cause(s)* • Add HCL • Probiotics &/or enzymes • Adjust diet
HEARTBURN, acid reflux **(GERD),** indigestion	• Excess stomach acid (HCL) • Low stomach acid (HCL) • Antacids overuse • Food sensitivities / allergies • Drug side effect • Muscle malfunction • Hiatal hernia • Low saliva *See Dry Mouth in Ch 8.*	*Conduct tests* • Elimination diet • Food allergies • GI exam *Address the cause(s)* • Add HCL • Physical therapy • Alternative drug • Avoid antacids
SLOW METABOLISM	• Low B vitamins • Low thyroid • Sedentary lifestyle	*Conduct tests* • Micronutrients • Thyroid function *Address the cause(s)* • B vitamins, esp. B12 & folate (folic acid) • Thyroid therapy • Increase exercise, esp. weight-bearing

Weight & Digestion (cont.)

PROBLEM	COMMON CAUSES	POSSIBLE SOLUTIONS
GAS	• Food allergies/ sensitivities • Low stomach acid (HCL) • Low digestive enzymes • Excess fiber in diet	*Conduct tests* • Elimination diet • Food allergies *Address the cause(s)* • Elimination/rotation diet • Add HCL • Probiotics &/or digestive enzymes • Decrease dietary fiber
CONSTIPATION	• Dehydration • Underactive thyroid • Nutritional deficiencies • Sex hormone imbalance • Drug side effect	*Conduct tests* • Thyroid hormones • Micronutrients • Sex hormones *Address the cause(s)* • Increase fluid intake • Thyroid therapy • Nutritional therapy • Add/balance sex hormones • Alternative drug *Address the symptoms* • High fiber diet • Prunes • Senna tea

Weight & Digestion (cont.)

PROBLEM	COMMON CAUSES	POSSIBLE SOLUTIONS
DIARRHEA	• Low gut bacteria • Nutritional deficiencies • Food allergies/ sensitivities • Lactose intolerance • Stress • *H. pylori* bacteria	***Conduct tests*** • Micronutrients • Food allergies • *H. pylori* ***Address the cause(s)*** • Probiotics • Nutritional therapy • Rotation diet • Lactase enzyme supplements • Antibiotics plus Pepto Bismol ***Address the symptoms*** • Anti-diarrhea drugs
STOMACH ULCER	• *H. pylori* bacteria • Excess stomach acid (rarely) • Drug side effect (esp. osteoporosis drugs) • Parasites • Stress	***Conduct tests*** • *H. pylori* • Parasites ***Address the cause(s)*** • Antibiotics plus Pepto Bismol • Alternative drug • Parasite cleanse • Reduce stress ***Address the symptoms*** • Bland diet

11 | Conditions & Diagnoses

This chapter differs from the previous chapters because here you have already identified a condition or diagnosis, whether on your own or through a physician.

Because you are probably familiar with the conventional solutions, we will cover only those complementary treatments and preventive measures your doctor may *not* mention.

CONDITION / DIAGNOSIS	COMPLEMENTARY SOLUTIONS
ADRENAL FATIGUE	• Adrenal support therapy • Reduce stress
ALS / Lou Gehrig's	• Add/balance sex hormones (esp. progesterone) • Nutritional therapy • Add estrogen • Eliminate excitotoxins (like MSG), and detox
ALZHEIMER'S	• Add testosterone (if low) • Vitamin D3 • Add estrogen, eliminate excitotoxins (like MSG), and detox
ASTROCYTOMA (type of brain tumor)	• Eliminate excitotoxins (especially aspartame), detox, and add estrogen

Conditions & Diagnoses (cont.)

CONDITION / DIAGNOSIS	COMPLEMENTARY SOLUTIONS
AUTOIMMUNE DISEASES (e.g., rheumatoid arthritis, MS, fibromyalgia, etc.)	▪ Add progesterone &/ or pregnenolone ▪ Vitamin D3 ▪ Nutritional therapy ▪ Elimination/rotation diet ▪ Probiotics
CANCER	▪ Vitamin D3 & other antioxidants ▪ Broccoli etc. (improve 2/16 ratio of good-to-bad estrogen breakdown molecules) ▪ Tagamet (cimetidine) ▪ Add/balance sex hormones
CHRONIC FATIGUE	▪ *See Fibromyalgia*
DIABETES (Type 2)	▪ Adrenal therapy ▪ Chromium ▪ Surgical bypass of duodenum & jejunum
FIBROIDS (uterine)	▪ Add progesterone
FIBROMYALGIA & CHRONIC FATIGUE	▪ High-dose IV vitamin therapy ▪ Add/balance sex hormones ▪ Treatment for thyroid resistance ▪ Nutritional therapy ▪ Growth hormone (GH)
GALLSTONES, gallbladder attacks	▪ Low fat diet ▪ Pancreatic enzymes, bile salts

Conditions & Diagnoses (cont.)

CONDITION / DIAGNOSIS	COMPLEMENTARY SOLUTIONS
HEART DISEASE, cardiovascular	▪ Add/balance sex hormones and/or growth hormone ▪ Nutritional therapy ▪ Omega 3 fish oils ▪ CoQ10/ubiquinol ▪ Vitamin D3, and B-complex (esp. B12, folate/folic acid, niacin) ▪ Antibiotics (for chronic infection) ▪ Inflammation-reducing supplements
HEAVY METAL TOXICITY/poisoning	▪ Cleanse/chelation
HIGH CHOLESTEROL (low HDL, high LDL & triglycerides	▪ Add/balance sex hormones ▪ High-dose omega-3 oils ▪ Exercise ▪ Nutritional therapy ▪ Liver cleanse
HYPERTENSION (high blood pressure)	▪ Balance potassium & calcium ▪ Vitamin D3 ▪ Hawthorn berry
IMMUNE DEFICIENCY *See Autoimmune Diseases*	▪ Elimination/rotation diet ▪ Vitamin D3, zinc, antioxidants ▪ Add progesterone and/or pregnenolone ▪ Adrenal therapy ▪ Probiotics ▪ *See Ch 3: Allergies & Immune Dysfunctions*

Conditions & Diagnoses (cont.)

CONDITION / DIAGNOSIS	COMPLEMENTARY SOLUTIONS
INFECTIONS (frequent)	▪ *See Immune Deficiency, above & Ch 3: Allergies & Immune Dysfunctions*
IRON EXCESS, hemochromatosis	▪ Reduce iron intake ▪ Donate blood (if not diagnosed with hemochromatosis) ▪ Balance sex hormones
LEAKY GUT SYNDROME	▪ Probiotics ▪ Elimination/rotation diet ▪ Cleanse (yeast/Candida, parasites)
LIVER DAMAGE/ DISORDERS	▪ Liver protection (milk thistle, bupleurum, etc.) ▪ Avoid toxins (drugs, alcohol)
MACULAR DEGENERATION (eyes)	*See Ch 8: Mouth, Eyes, Nose, Ears*
OSTEOPOROSIS	▪ Vitamin D3 ▪ Calcium, magnesium, protein ▪ Weight-bearing exercise ▪ pH balance ▪ Add/balance sex hormones
OVARIAN CYSTS, (PCOS)	▪ Reduce/balance testosterone ▪ Add/balance progesterone
PANCREATIC DISORDERS	▪ Diabetic diet ▪ Nutritional therapy

Conditions & Diagnoses (cont.)

CONDITION / DIAGNOSIS	COMPLEMENTARY SOLUTIONS
PARKINSON'S DISEASE	• Add testosterone • Add estrogen • Eliminate excitotoxins (MSG, aspartame, etc.) • Detox
SPASTIC COLON, irritable bowel	• Elimination/rotation diet
SURGERY, injury	• L glutamine (speed healing)
THYROID (overactive)	• Iodine
THYROID (underactive)	• Add/balance progesterone • Iodine
UTERINE PROLAPSE	• Add/balance sex hormones
VIRAL INFECTION (preventive)	• High dose vitamin C • Quercetin • Melatonin

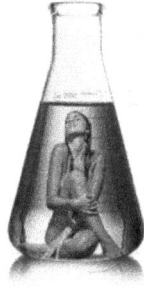

PART B: **TESTS**

YOUR TESTING INFORMATION

Use this page to make notes about testing, or list key results of tests you may have had.

_____

_____

_____

_____

_____

_____

_____

_____

_____

_____

_____

_____

_____

_____

_____

_____

_____

_____

_____

12| What You Need to Know About Testing

Smart women know that the war against aging is best fought *offensively*, by doing everything possible to *maintain* health, youthfulness and vitality before it is lost. And when they see that damage has already been done, they quickly seek out the best solutions to restore the balance nature intended.

Phenomenal women know that only by addressing the *causes* of aging and dysfunction can we truly maintain our bodies and minds in a state of optimal wellness.

In order to know what's going on inside the processes that keep you in top form, you may need tests.

Your trusted healthcare advisors will typically identify the need for a given test, and will order it and interpret its results for you. Therefore, this chapter will focus primarily on what you need to know about the different types of tests you might encounter in your quest for youthful wellness and vibrancy.

Some tests are conducted entirely by healthcare or laboratory professionals. Others may require your involvement to varying degrees.

Certain tests are available that you can order and/or perform on your own, independent of your healthcare advisors. These may allow you to observe and monitor ongoing conditions more often than your doctor would normally require. This practice can provide useful information to you and your healthcare team. However, if you get testing done on your own, be sure to give your doctors copies of all the results for their records.

Types of Tests

There are many types of tests that can help shine a light on the real cause of what's bothering you. And, in a best-case scenario, they can even help catch dysfunctions before they do any lasting damage.

Useful tests include:

- Blood/serum
- Saliva
- Urine
- Stool
- Hair
- Imaging
- Dietary
- Allergy
- Nerve

BLOOD/SERUM TESTS

We've all had blood tests, so there's not much you don't know about them...with a few notable exceptions.

FREE/UNBOUND HORMONES

For some crazy reason, nature tends to lock up (bind) a large percentage of our sex hormones. So it's important to find out how much of the total amount in your body is actually *available* (*free* or unbound) for use by your tissues.

There are two ways to determine your free hormone levels:

- The **direct** method measures the actual amount of the free portion of a given hormone in your blood
- The **calculation** method measures the *total* amount of hormone circulating in your blood, then *estimates* the free amount according to the average free-to-total proportion.

Because a number of conditions can throw off the expected ratio of free-to-total hormone levels, the calculation method may not always yield an accurate picture. So be sure your doctor is using the direct method when testing hormones via blood.

BIO-IDENTICAL HORMONES VS. HORSE OR SYNTHETIC HORMONES

If you are taking hormones (estrogen, progesterone, testosterone or thyroid) it's important to understand that standard blood tests can only measure the amount of *human or bio-identical* (chemically identical to human) hormones in your bloodstream.

So if you take Premarin, for example, you may have a lot of very potent estrogens in your body, but most of these are *horse estrogens* and won't show up on your blood test, which is looking for human or bio-identical estrogens.

Similarly, if you are taking a synthetic (bio-deviant) progesterone, testosterone or thyroid substitute, your blood tests may still show your hormone levels are low (even when they aren't) because the tests are only able to measure human and bio-identical forms of those hormones.

On the other hand, if you are taking a bio-identical hormone such as estradiol, progesterone, or even Armour thyroid, your blood tests *will* recognize the supplements. That's because they look exactly like the ones nature makes in your body, even though the hormone may be made from yams or, in the case of Armour thyroid, from *pig* thyroid glands.

As it happens, nature designed pigs and humans to operate on the exact same thyroid hormones in roughly the same proportions. Therefore, pig thyroid hormones are *bio-identical* to those in humans and will be reflected in your thyroid tests.

SALIVA TESTS

Many healthcare practitioners believe that measuring free hormones in saliva is much more accurate than blood tests.

If your doctor or healthcare advisor recommends a saliva test, you should know that this is a test you will do at home and will then mail it back to a lab in a prepaid box or envelope.

In some cases only one test tube of saliva will be needed. In others—when testing cortisol for adrenal function, for example—you may have multiple tubes for collections at specific times of day.

Each kit typically contains:

- 1 or more sealable test tubes for the collection of saliva (spit)
- Labels for the tubes
- A zippered biohazard bag to put the tubes in for mailing
- An absorbent pad to go inside the biohazard bag
- Forms to be completed and mailed back with the samples
- A box for mailing
- A prepaid mailing label and/or outer mailing bag

You will also need a thin-point permanent marker or black pen to label your tubes.

Because not all labs' kits include clear instructions, here are a few tips that can help:

- Fill out the forms when you get the kit. You may also want to copy the completed forms for your records.

- Pick a day to do your test when you will be at home or with access to a refrigerator, and can have a certain amount of privacy for the collections.

- Make notes in a journal or separate piece of paper for yourself showing where you were in your cycle or in your treatment regimen (especially if you are monitoring the effects of that regimen on blood/saliva levels) at the time of the test.

- Wait until after you've collected each sample to apply its label. (Otherwise, the label may obscure a measuring line.)

- For the day's first collection (before eating), rinse your mouth with cool water, then begin spitting saliva into the tube. Fill the tube according to directions. (Foam doesn't count, only liquid.) If you have trouble generating saliva, think of lemons, or even cut a lemon open and smell it.

- Seal and label the tube and, if you aren't ready to mail it out yet, put it in a baggie in the freezer.

- For each subsequent sample during the day, wait at least an hour after the previous meal, then rinse your mouth with water and collect the saliva sample. Freeze it with the others, if necessary.

- When you have all the samples collected and are ready to mail them out, put the tubes and the pad inside the biohazard bag and zip it up.

- Next, complete the forms (if not already done) and put them inside the mailing box with the biohazard bag full of tubes.

- Close/seal the box inside the mailing bag (if there is one), and put the prepaid mailing/shipping label on the outside of the bag or box (if no bag).

- Follow the shipping/mailing instructions (which may use US Postal Service, UPS, or other method). In some cases you can call the carrier for a pickup or drop the package off at an authorized location.

- In most cases the results will be sent to your healthcare advisor. However, if you've ordered the kit yourself, the results will come directly to you.

URINE TESTS

There are few mysteries about urine tests. We've all done them. However, there are a few secrets you might not be aware of.

PH BALANCE

Your body's fluids generally prefer to maintain fairly neutral conditions, with a pH of around 7.4, which is just slightly to the alkaline (non-acid) side of neutral.

If the pH is off too far to either side, it indicates that something is wrong. And if you don't adjust it, your body may fail to absorb nutrients, screen out toxins and repair damaged cells.

An easy way to check your pH balance uses a simple dipstick, like the litmus paper you experimented with in science class. Some dipsticks are more detailed than others.

Unlike the simple pink/blue litmus papers, the ones used for testing urine (or saliva) pH may have a range of colors. But they all work the same way: you dip them into the fluid you are testing, then compare the color you get with the chart in the kit.

See Chapter 21 for more about pH balance and bone health.

MENOPAUSE DIPSTICK TEST

As you will discover in Chapter 14, there is one brain hormone, called FSH, that begins to "yell" when your estrogen is too low.

During your reproductive years, it yells (or peaks) for just a brief time in the middle of each menstrual month in order to get your estrogen to spike, forcing the matured egg off the ovary at ovulation.

But when you're no longer ovulating, no longer responding to your brain's demands, your FSH keeps yelling (remains high).

Today, there are over-the-counter dipstick tests, like pregnancy tests, to help you look for sustained high levels of FSH indicating that you may be hormonally menopausal.

You will need to perform multiple tests at different times of the month, possibly during multiple months in order to be sure you are no longer fertile (because FSH will naturally be high during the hours around ovulation). What's more significant is a high FSH reading around day 6 or day 22 of your cycle when FSH should be low again.

STOOL TESTS

Icky as they seem, stool (feces/poop) tests can be quite valuable, especially in identifying bacteria or parasites that may have taken up residence in your gut. They are also helpful in diagnosing certain food sensitivities and in finding "occult" blood that could be an early indicator of colon cancer.

Like the saliva tests, many stool tests are done at home and must be mailed back to the lab using a prepaid package. *(See Saliva Tests.)*

HAIR TESTS

Like the rings of a tree, your slow-growing hair provides a relative history of your exposure to a variety of substances.

If warranted, your healthcare advisor may suggest a hair test to look for heavy metal (aluminum, mercury, arsenic, lead, etc.) toxicities.

You may do this test at your healthcare advisor's office. If you are asked to do it at home, you will be required to snip a few hairs close to the scalp, then trim them and mail them to the lab in a prepaid mailer.

NOTE: Be aware that hair analysis *alone* cannot accurately diagnose toxicities and vitamin deficiencies.

X-RAYS AND IMAGING TESTS

Most of us are familiar with the most common imaging tests: conventional x-rays, CTs, MRIs, mammograms, sonograms and bone density scans.

They all have their plusses and minuses, but one stands out as worthy of a bit more discussion: *CT scans.*

CT SCANS USE HIGH-DOSE X-RAYS

We tend to think of CTs as being safer than common x-rays. But that couldn't be further from the truth. CT scans are simply longer-duration, more-detailed, three-dimensional x-rays. Just one CT scan can expose you to extremely high doses of x-rays.

To put it into perspective:

- A normal chest x-ray exposes you to about 10 millirem (mrem).
- Each year, you'll get about 100-300 mrem from normal background radiation in the environment.
- Exposure from a mammogram is around 300 mrem.
- A **chest CT** exposes you to **580 mrem** (58 chest x-rays).
- A **virtual colonoscopy** (CT) can expose you to some **800 mrem** (80 chest x-rays)
- And just one cardiac CT angiogram or a barium enema CT can expose you to around **1300-1500 mrem** (or up to 150 chest x-rays).

While these can tests can be extraordinarily valuable when your doctors need to see inside you, their radiation can be damaging.

Remember: This is the kind of radiation that can mutate the DNA in your cells. The higher the dose or the more often you have the tests, the more mutated cells your overworked immune system has to round up and kill—and the more likely it is that a gang of them will evade your defenses to start growing a cancer.

So don't get these kinds of tests unless you *really* need them.

ALLERGY TESTS

For those who suffer the classic symptoms of allergies —
sneezing, runny nose, itchy eyes — it's easy to recognize the need
for a treatment.

But many of us exhibit our allergies in less obvious ways. So if
you are having certain issues that seem to defy conventional
treatments, it may be helpful to ask whether your symptoms
might be related to allergies.

TRADITIONAL ALLERGY TESTS

Allergies are traditionally diagnosed using a series of skin tests.
These tests measure IgE antibodies, which will produce an
almost immediate reaction.

In the first series, a nurse or technician may create a grid of little
scratches or pinpricks on your back, with each prick containing a
certain type of allergen or class of allergens.

In the second type of test, the technician injects a little bubble of
each allergen just under your skin.

In both tests, your reaction (redness in the skin around the site)
tells the allergist what you are allergic to and to what degree.

DIETARY ALLERGIES/SENSITIVITIES TESTS

Food sensitivities may be tested either by trying the elimination
diet or by using an IgG blood test.

While traditional allergies are tested by measuring the IgE
antibodies that produce immediate reactions, food testing looks
for IgG antibodies, which can trigger *delayed* reactions. Because
you may not react to a troublesome food for hours or days, it
may be hard to connect the reaction with a given food without
an IgG test.

When testing for food sensitivities by elimination, you will typically have to remove all but the most harmless foods from your diet until your symptoms go away or ease up. Then you can add back one type of food at a time to see if your symptoms return. As long as your symptoms do not return, you can keep adding foods back into your diet.

Once you discover a food that triggers the symptoms again, you may have to eliminate it and wait until your symptoms subside before continuing to add more new foods.

The whole process of identifying foods (and drinks) you are allergic/sensitive to can take days or even weeks.

Tests Results

When you see the results of a given test, especially hormone tests, you may notice that there are several columns. The most important are:

- Your actual values
- Flags for high/low values
- Reference ranges

ACTUAL VALUES & FLAGS

When you look at your hormone levels in test reports, note whether these reflect *total* or *free* hormones. And if a given value reflects the amount of free or unbound hormone, ask whether it was measured directly or was calculated.

The *flags* column alerts you to note those actual values that are above or below the reference ranges.

REFERENCE RANGE

The *reference range* for each item indicates the level of that hormone (or other substance) that is considered to be within the "normal" range.

BEWARE OF THE "NORMAL" MISINTERPRETATION

Because most peri- and post-menopausal women naturally have low and imbalanced hormones, the reference ranges on hormone lab tests will invariably indicate that any low hormones are perfectly "normal."

Similarly, your mechanic may tell you that it's *normal* for your car to run low on oil after several thousand miles of driving. But he will also tell you that if you don't replace the oil, your engine will seize up and die.

Sadly, the same logic may not always be applied to humans, especially when it comes to sex hormones.

The fact is that we should always measure a substance according to *optimal values*, not the randomly occurring normal ranges. And we should supplement those substances when necessary to achieve optimal levels unless there are compelling medical reasons not to.

UNITS OF MEASURE

If you are keeping track of test results from a number of different sources or are comparing one item to another, be sure to pay attention to the units of measure.

One hormone may be measured in picograms per milliliters (pg/mL), while another is in nanograms per milliliter (ng/mL). Still other substances may be measured in international units (IUs), or picomoles per liter (pmol/L).

It's important to compare any before/after test results *in the same units of measure*, (apple to apples), even if you have to convert one or more of the values (e.g., pg/mL to pmol/L) to get them all into the same units.

VARIATIONS BETWEEN LABS

Be aware that results can differ between labs and even within the same lab at different times of day.

Use lab results as *relative measures* of ratios and of variations, not as absolutes.

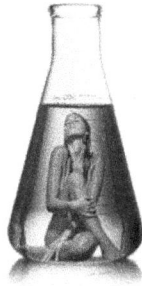

PART C: **HEALTH PROCESSES**

WELLNESS NOTES

Use this page to make notes about the various health processes
and how your body is supposed to work under optimal
conditions.

_____

_____

_____

_____

_____

_____

_____

_____

_____

_____

_____

_____

_____

_____

_____

_____

_____

_____

_____

_____

_____

13 | Health Processes

Your youthfulness and vibrancy depend on the optimal functioning of many interconnected systems. An imbalance or dysfunction in one can throw off any number of other, seemingly unrelated, processes.

So it is important to know how these processes are supposed to work, how they interact with one another, and how the various organs and glands keep everything running.

The four key processes are:

- **Hormonal**
- **Nutritional**
- **Nervous system/communication**
- **Purification (immune and detoxification)**

Each process depends upon the others in order to do its job. For example:

➤ To make many of your hormones you need cholesterol, the majority of which is made in your liver (only a small portion comes from food).

➤ Your nutritional processes must break down that food to release its nutrients into your bloodstream.

➤ The nervous system relays signals from your body to the brain telling it that a given hormone is low and to trigger the release of more of that hormone from its source glands.

➤ The hormones circulate to targeted tissues, turning on/off specific functions.

> ➤ And finally the liver mops up the leftover cholesterol, breaks it down and pushes it out into the intestines for removal along with toxins and other wastes.

And what happens when these intricately coordinated events don't happen as they should?

> ➤ If something is wrong with your digestive system, you may not be getting the proper nutrients from food.

> ➤ If your hormone-making machinery has shut down or has been removed, or if you don't have the necessary raw materials to make hormones, the functions of other systems will be compromised.

> ➤ If your nerves are kinked or compressed, signals between the brain and body may be lost or garbled.

> ➤ And if your immune and detoxification systems aren't effectively disabling threats and taking out the trash on a regular basis, nothing else will matter because disease processes will take control of your body.

So you see how complex and interconnected our systems are. This is why specialists may fail to see the bigger picture or why narrowly focused treatments may only address the *symptoms* rather then resolving or preventing the *cause*.

The goal of this book is to help you and your healthcare team see The Big Picture—to evaluate your wellness or dysfunction from a holistic point of view, and to develop a preventive program or remediation therapy that addresses your whole body and your whole life experience.

14 | Hormonal/Endocrine Processes

Hormones are truly the "magic potions" we rely on every day to make our bodies do what they are supposed to do.

- They make us grow and direct that growth toward male or female characteristics.

- They make us feel hungry/full, sleepy/alert, sexy, happy, assertive or nurturing.

- They make sure we have the fuel we need to get up in the morning, to work, think and remember, and to respond to emergencies. And they put us to sleep at night.

- They help us burn off the food we eat and use nutrients to build bones and muscles and other tissues.

- They help us make babies and keep our systems safely balanced when we're not making babies.

- They control things like blood pressure, kidney function and the levels of various substances in the blood.

- They attack invaders and heal our wounds.

- And they make defective cells commit suicide so they can't turn into cancers.

Hormones literally make us who we are. If you don't believe it, consider how children change when they go through puberty. Think about how women change during pregnancy or at menopause.

And these are only the most obvious hormonal influences. The majority of our hormones go about their work without ever being noticed...until something goes wrong.

Key Hormones

These are some of the most important hormones and the jobs they do:

- **Aldosterone** (maintains blood pressure, controls fluid flow in kidneys)
- **Calcitonin/calcitriol/vitamin D** (builds bone, boosts immune system)
- **Cortisol and adrenalin/epinephrine** (release energy, increase heart rate, narrow blood vessels, open airways, balance water and salt, regulate breakdown of foods, reduce inflammation)
- **DHEA** (supports brain function, produces testosterone)
- **Eicosanoids** *hormone-like substances such as prostaglandins, leukotrienes, thromboxanes* (stimulate inflammation, pain and swelling in response to threats to your body)
- **Endorphins** (reduce pain, promote feeling of wellbeing)
- **Follicle-stimulating hormone/ FSH** (matures eggs)
- **Gastrin** (releases stomach acid)
- **Ghrelin** (stimulates appetite, stimulates growth hormone)
- **Glucose/blood sugar** (the primary source of everyday fuel for virtually all cells)
- **Growth hormone** (stimulates growth and cell division, repairs tissues, maintains bones, brain, muscle, skin, hair, nails)
- **Histamine** (stimulates stomach acid)
- **Insulin** (regulates blood sugar, produces triglycerides)
- **Leptin** (decreases appetite, increases metabolism)
- **Melatonin** (promotes sleep and cellular repair, suppresses estrogen production overnight)
- **Oxytocin** (stimulates bonding emotions, release of breast milk, triggers orgasm and labor contractions of the uterus)

- **Parathyroid** (increases blood calcium, activates vitamin D, reduces anxiety, promotes feelings of wellbeing)
- **Prolactin** (produces breast milk, promotes feelings of satisfaction after sex)
- **Serotonin** (controls mood, appetite, promotes sleep)
- **Thyroid hormones** (control metabolism, body temperature)
- **Thyroid stimulating hormone** (triggers release of thyroid hormones)

And then there are the sex hormones. Although they do play a prominent role in sex and reproduction, they also perform critical jobs in non-reproductive functions.

- **Estrogens.** *(E1/estrone, E2/estradiol, E3/estriol)* Develop female sex traits, stimulate cell division and enable reproduction, build milk-secreting glands in the breast, slow bone loss, maintain tissue elasticity and retain fluid/moisture, *reduce* muscle mass, promote a mellow and nurturing mood, retain fat (for emergencies), maintain heart health, support brain function.

- **Progesterone.** Enables reproduction, modifies uterine lining, moderates immune system so mom's body doesn't reject baby, builds ducts in breast to drain milk, balances estrogen effects, builds bone and muscle, promotes fat burning, releases fluid from tissues, stabilizes blood sugar, supports thyroid function, delivers oxygen to cells, elevates mood, supports brain function and sex drive.

- **Testosterone.** Stimulates sexual fantasy and desire/arousal, builds bone and muscle, maintains heart and brain function, elevates mood, promotes assertiveness.

Organs and Glands

The most significant organs in the endocrine or hormonal system are the pituitary, pineal, hypothalamus, thyroid, adrenals, kidneys, pancreas, and ovaries.

Organs Involved in Hormonal/Endocrine Processes

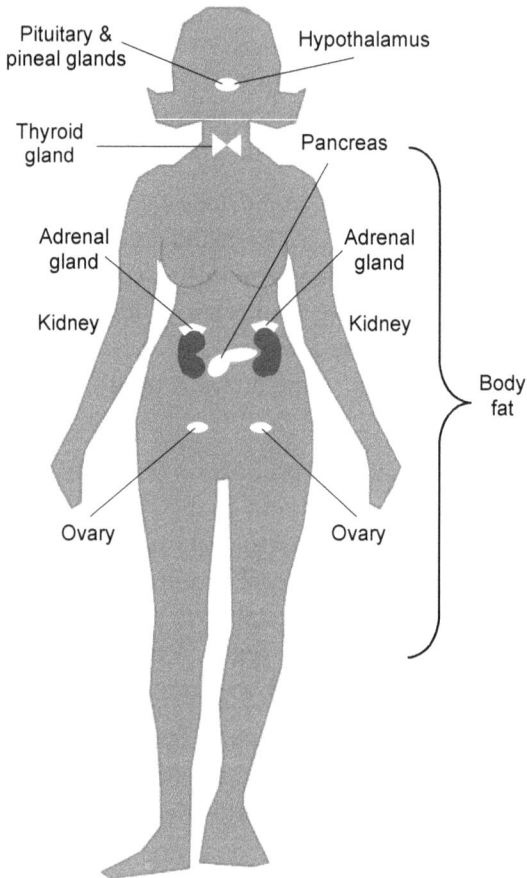

And as you can see from the diagram above, body fat also plays an important role in these processes as well. Let's find out more about these key organs and glands.

ADRENAL GLANDS

The two adrenal glands sit on top of each kidney.

Their primary role is to produce the **stress hormones cortisol and adrenalin (epinephrine)**. They produce the hormone **aldosterone** to **regulate blood pressure** and **electrolyte balance** and maintain **kidney function**. They help **balance blood sugar** and decrease inflammation by releasing the body's **natural anti-inflammatory hormone (cortisol)**.

They also produce about half of your normal supply of **testosterone and DHEA**, serve as a **backup source** of **estradiol (estrogen)**, and provide a tiny amount of **progesterone**.

Cortisol stimulates your appetite, improves digestion, stimulates the brain, heart, lungs and muscles, increases circulation, and, like the synthetic steroids the doctor may give you, this natural steroid reduces inflammation and can improve mobility in stiff joints.

The stress hormones were designed to give you extra fuel to respond to emergencies. They make your heart race and they mobilize energy from your cells. If you have a true emergency (as nature imagined), your body will also be racing to escape or cope with danger. This typically would burn off the cortisol and adrenalin.

But in the modern world, we often raise our stress hormone levels just worrying about issues in our lives. Our bodies release the same hormones, but instead of running or climbing a tree in response, we often just sit in front of the TV or computer, or eat comfort food (high carb junk). That cortisol remains in the blood, decreasing the ability of our cells to respond to insulin (triggering insulin resistance). And the adrenalin lingers to keep our pulse racing and to prevent restful sleep.

In the short term, cortisol will give you a boost of energy. But over time, too much stress (that is, too much cortisol and/or adrenalin) weakens your immune system, reducing your infection-fighting white blood cell count and making you more vulnerable to infection. It interferes with the repairs that should take place during sleep, reduces your production of DHEA, may increase allergies, and will almost certainly leave you feeling exhausted.

Signs of excess cortisol can include:

- Swollen tissues
- Low blood pressure
- Hair loss (especially from the top of your head)
- Sugar/salt cravings
- Sluggish digestion, constipation
- Allergies, eczema
- Confusion
- Difficulty with sexual arousal

ADRENAL FATIGUE

Adrenal fatigue occurs when the adrenals are kept on high alert, responding to everyday stresses for an extended period. These stressors can be anything the body perceives as an emergency and can include:

- Emotional stress
- Poor nutrition
- Insomnia, inadequate sleep
- Illness, injury

Your adrenals normally make between 20 and 30 mg of cortisol each day. If you are *above* that level, your adrenals are probably overstressed, pumping out high levels of cortisol to fuel all your perceived emergencies.

If your cortisol is *below* normal, you are probably in an advanced phase of adrenal fatigue in which the glands are so worn out they can no longer supply even a normal amount of cortisol.

There are 4 stages of adrenal fatigue:

- **STAGE 1: Alarm Reaction.** In this stage, the adrenals are doing what they were designed to do: mobilize your emergency energy/fuel sources by releasing extra cortisol and/or adrenalin. This response is initiated by the pituitary's release of ACTH, a messenger hormone, which then shuts off again when the brain learns that the adrenal hormone levels have increased.

- **STAGE 2: Resistance Response.** When you remain stressed for an extended time, your adrenals eventually become unable to produce sustained high levels of cortisol. You begin to feel more tired in the morning and during the day. And with your cortisol supplies running low, your body begins to convert more and more of the parent hormone, pregnenolone, into cortisol (a phenomenon sometimes called "pregnenolone steal"), instead of using it to make progesterone, estrogen and testosterone.

- **STAGE 3: Exhaustion.** In this stage, your pituitary is "screaming" for more cortisol by releasing ACTH, but the adrenals simply can't produce enough to shut off that demand signal in the brain. As a side effect, the adrenals fail to produce their share of the sex hormones estrogen, testosterone, and that tiny bit of progesterone, so those levels drop as well.

- **STAGE 4: Failure.** If the adrenals completely fail and you do not replace their hormones, you can die.

WHAT YOU NEED TO KNOW ABOUT CORTISOL

Although cortisol is a handy hormone to have when you need to cram for finals or get that mission-critical 200-page report out the door before tomorrow morning, you pay a price for its benefits.

Think of it this way: If you are trapped in a cabin under an avalanche of snow, you will burn everything you can find—including the furniture—to keep from freezing to death until rescuers arrive. But you wouldn't want to do that on a regular basis. There are better, smarter ways to heat the house on a day-to-day basis.

Similarly, there are other, more effective, sources of fuel (primarily glucose) stored away in fat and muscle cells that are intended for your daily use and replenishment.

Because priorities change in emergencies, your body understands that it might have to "burn the furniture" to release the necessary energy to keep you alive. So it lets cortisol burn cells from wherever it finds them: your lungs, liver, heart, kidneys, muscles, skin, or even your brain. It doesn't care.

That's why it is so **critically important to lower the stress in your life in order to rejuvenate and restore your body to optimal performance**. Nothing else will matter if you stress your body by worrying over every issue, eating junk food, skipping meals, ingesting toxins or cheating on sleep.

BODY FAT

It may seem odd to mention fat as a source of hormones, but fat actually has the ability to convert other hormones into estrogen. So for the purpose of understanding how hormones are made, it's important to consider the role of fat in altering hormone levels and balances.

HYPOTHALAMUS GLAND

Sitting right next to the pituitary gland, the **hypothalamus controls** your **circadian rhythm** of sleeping and waking. And it manages many of the body's functions like **temperature regulation and sweating, blood pressure, heart rate, shivering, fluid retention, electrolyte balance, hunger/full signals,** stomach secretions, immune response, and even maternal feelings and behaviors.

It is also responsible for your response to smells, especially those of pheromones that are involved in sexual attraction.

Because the hypothalamus and pituitary are so close, both physically and functionally, when your ovarian hormone levels drop and the pituitary goes into overdrive trying to compensate, the functions of the hypothalamus can also be disrupted, causing some of those bothersome symptoms like hot flashes, night sweats and heart palpitations.

KIDNEYS

The kidneys are located a few inches above your waist on either side of your body.

In addition to filtering out waste products, the kidneys help maintain your body's acid-base balance (keeping it relatively neutral at an ideal pH of about 7.3), and help maintain your electrolyte balance.

Your kidneys also play an critical role in maintaining your blood pressure.

OVARIES

The ovaries are located on either side of the pelvis at the end of the two fallopian tubes that direct eggs into the uterus.

The ovaries produce three key hormones:
- Estrogen (E1/estrone, E2/estradiol, and E3/estriol)
- Testosterone
- Progesterone (only after ovulation)

During reproductive years, your ovaries supply about half your testosterone, 65% of your estrogen, and 90% of your progesterone.

That's why, when your ovaries shut down at menopause, you may end up with not just *low* hormones but dangerously *imbalanced* hormones.

PANCREAS

The pancreas is a spongy organ about the size of a banana, located between the stomach and the small intestine.

Its two most important jobs are to **secrete digestive enzymes** to break down carbohydrates, fats and proteins in your food, and to **produce insulin to regulate your blood sugar**.

PINEAL GLAND

Located deep in the brain, this tiny gland (the size of a grain of rice) is a powerhouse when it comes to helping us get to **sleep**.

It secretes the hormone **melatonin** when we are in darkness.

It is important to note that those of us who sleep with the TV on or with night lights and glowing clocks in the bedroom may not be getting the most beneficial sleep. Research has shown that even a small amount of light (especially blue light) will suppress the brain's production of sleep-promoting melatonin and turn on the production of energy-driving cortisol.

PITUITARY GLAND

This gland lies just above the roof of your mouth. It hangs down from the base of the brain like a small pea in a sack.

The pituitary is considered the **endocrine system's "master gland"** because it **controls** the activity of many other glands and organs, including the **brain, thyroid, breasts, kidneys, adrenals, ovaries, uterus, bones and muscle**.

The pituitary gland secretes a number of important hormones including:

- **Growth hormone** (GH)
- **Thyroid stimulating hormone** (TSH)
- **Follicle stimulating hormone** (FSH)
- **Prolactin**
- **Endorphins**
- **Oxytocin**
- **ACTH** (adrenal stimulating hormone)

The pituitary supplies a number of our important **"feel good" hormones** like endorphins, oxytocin and prolactin.

If the pituitary is not functioning properly or is overactive because of a tumor, it can throw off any number of systems.

In particular, when the pituitary is overactive during perimenopause, it can irritate its neighbor, the hypothalamus, which can result in wild fluctuations of body temperature and heart rate. *(See Hypothalamus.)*

THYROID GLAND

Like a thick bowtie, the thyroid gland lies at the base of the neck and it is controlled by the pituitary. It produces three key hormones: T3, T4 and calcitonin. Virtually every cell in your body needs thyroid hormones.

The thyroid's most important job is to **regulate your metabolism to help you burn calories.** And its hormones are important for **proper growth and development.** It also plays a role in regulating **calcium** levels in your body and its use of **vitamin D.**

Iodine is important for the proper functioning of the thyroid gland, so those who don't eat a lot of seafood may need to use iodized salt or take iodine supplements.

THYROID DYSFUNCTION

It's important to note that many symptoms of high thyroid (*hyper*thyroid) hormone levels are the same as those of low (*hypo*thyroid) thyroid levels (*and* sex hormone imbalances).

SYMPTOMS OF THYROID DYSFUNCTION	Low T	Hi T
Fatigue & weakness	x	x
Dry, coarse skin	x	x
Hair loss	x	x
Brain fog, forgetfulness	x	x
Nervousness, shaking	x	x
Immune system dysfunction	x	x
Infertility	x	x
Insomnia (*most common with high thyroid*)	x	x
Depression (*with or without anxiety*)	x	
Anxiety (*with or without depression*)		x
Weight gain, difficulty losing weight	x	
Weight loss, difficulty gaining weight		x
Low temperature (*cold intolerance*), cold hands/feet	x	
High temperature (*heat intolerance*), warm hands/feet		x
Clammy skin		x
Loss of outer third of eyebrows	x	
Constipation	x	
Frequent bowel movements		x
Heavy menstrual periods	x	
Light menstrual periods		x
General muscle / joint pain, cramps, stiffness	x	
Carpal/tarsal (hand/foot) tunnel syndrome, tendonitis	x	
Trouble climbing stairs, gripping, reaching overhead		x
High cholesterol levels unresponsive to treatment	x	
Unusually low cholesterol levels		x

THYROID TESTING

It can be tricky to get an accurate view of your thyroid function. That's why your healthcare advisors may want to look at your thyroid hormones from a number of perspectives. They may order blood tests including:

- T3 (total)
- T4 (total)
- T3 uptake
- Reverse T3
- TSH
- Free T3 and T4
- T7 (free thyroxine index)
- Thyroid antibodies

And they may order a urine test for iodine as well.

THYROID AND IODINE

Because *iodine is essential to thyroid function*, most of us need to use iodized salt or take iodine supplements to support the thyroid (unless we eat *a lot* of seafood). Without iodine, our mental abilities and physiological growth processes can be severely retarded.

Iodine deficiency is the most common cause of thyroid dysfunction. However, **low progesterone** levels can also suppress thyroid function. So if you suspect thyroid problems, be sure to test your progesterone as well.

Be aware that your thyroid needs just the right amount of iodine. Too little and the thyroid can't make its critical hormones. Too much and it blocks the thyroid from making its hormones. It can even trigger an autoimmune response.

So once again, it's all about balance.

Hormones and Receptors

It's important that you understand *how hormones get into the cells* of your body to do their jobs. And it's equally important that you understand *how those hormones get back out of your cells* so they can be flushed away after they're done.

Each of your cells have little docking stations, like many keyholes in a door. And your hormone molecules have keys.

The keys on your hormone molecules allow them to dock with cells and turn on certain functions the cell is capable of performing. A given cell might have many different keyholes, or *receptors*, that allow a number of different hormones to dock with the cell and turn on various functions.

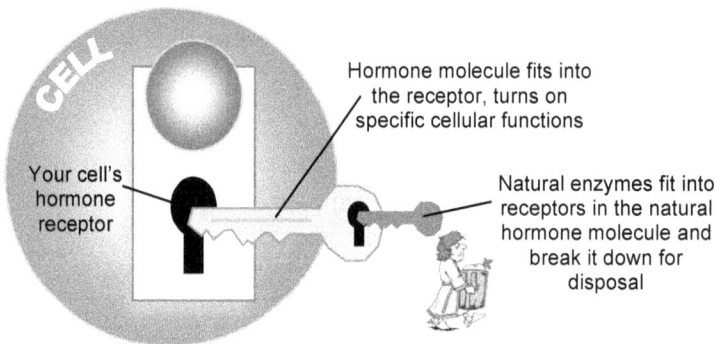

Hormone molecule fits into the receptor, turns on specific cellular functions

Your cell's hormone receptor

Natural enzymes fit into receptors in the natural hormone molecule and break it down for disposal

But those hormone molecules shouldn't stay in your cells indefinitely or the cells couldn't rest. So hormone molecules have keyholes of their own. While one end of the molecule (the key) docks with the cell's receptor (keyhole), the other end of the hormone molecule has a receptor (keyhole) of its own that an enzyme with the right key can dock with and begin to break down that hormone molecule so it can be flushed out of your body.

This lock-and-key process becomes especially important when we talk about *bio-identical* (chemically identical to your natural hormones) and *bio-deviant* (chemically alien to your body) hormones.

You've already learned that bio-identical hormones will show up in your hormone tests, while alien/bio-deviant hormones won't.

The other, much more important, point is that while bio-identical and natural human hormones can be broken down efficiently by the enzymes your body makes, those human enzymes can't dock with alien/bio-deviant hormones (horse hormones, synthetic hormones, etc.). And so the alien hormones can remain stuck in your cells' receptors, overstimulating the cells, exaggerating their effects and creating dramatic, and potentially dangerous, imbalances.

That's one of the many reasons why bio-identical hormones are better for your body than bio-deviant hormones.

Women and Sex Hormones

A man's sex hormones will remain relatively consistent, gradually declining with age. But a woman's sex hormones fluctuate dramatically within each month in a relatively predictable pattern throughout her fertile years.

And while some of our sex hormones decline gradually, like a man's, our progesterone can drop like a rock, both during months when we do not ovulate, and after menopause (or hysterectomy) when we are producing virtually no progesterone at all.

Curiously, a post-menopausal woman may actually have *less* estrogen than a man of the same age because he has more testosterone that can be converted into estrogen in fat cells!

Relative Estrogen Levels by Age *(Men & Women)*

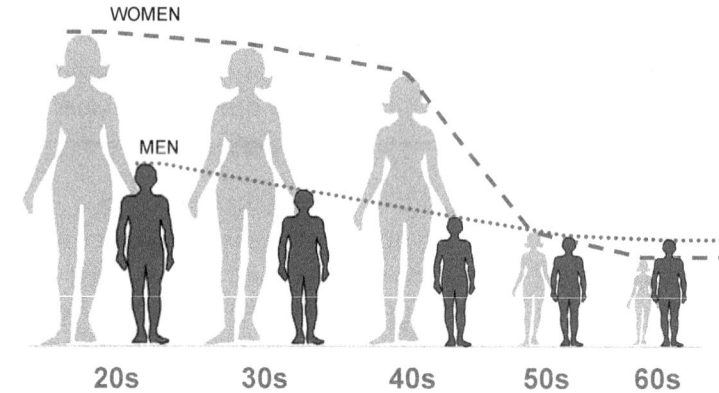

THE NORMAL MONTHLY CYCLE

When your reproductive system is working the way it's supposed to, your body spends roughly the first half of the month raising your estrogen levels.

- For the purposes of baby-making, **estrogen begins to rise** after your period, building up a nice cozy uterine lining and stimulating the ovaries to develop one or more eggs.

- Your ovaries and adrenal glands produce **testosterone** to **make you feel sexy**.

- The brain hormone, **FSH, spikes** in mid-month to **trigger ovulation**.

- **Estrogen reaches its peak** around the **middle of the month**, when **ovulation** occurs. That's when the matured egg pops out of the ovary and starts its journey down the fallopian tube toward the uterus where it hopes to meet a nice sperm and make a baby.

- Like the start and end of your period, the **actual day of ovulation can vary** considerably from month to month and among different women.

A Month WITH Ovulation

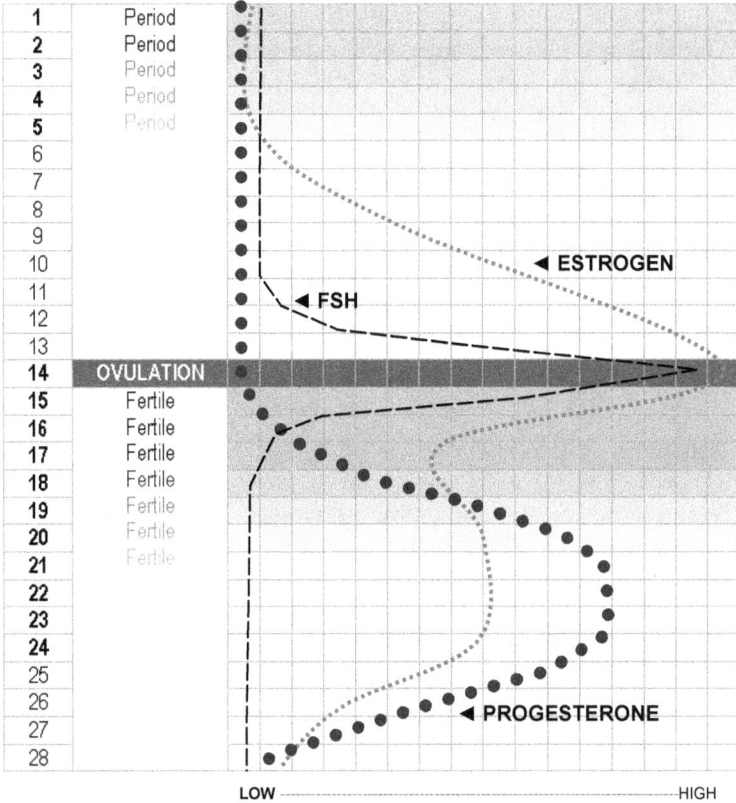

1	Period
2	Period
3	Period
4	Period
5	Period
6	
7	
8	
9	
10	
11	
12	
13	
14	OVULATION
15	Fertile
16	Fertile
17	Fertile
18	Fertile
19	Fertile
20	Fertile
21	Fertile
22	
23	
24	
25	
26	
27	
28	

◄ ESTROGEN

◄ FSH

◄ PROGESTERONE

LOW ────────────────────────────────────── HIGH

- As soon as the egg leaves the ovary, its empty nest (the **follicle) produces progesterone** for the next couple of weeks. That **softens the uterine lining** and makes it ready for implantation of the fertilized egg.

- **Progesterone** should be between **35 and 75 times higher than** your **estrogen** levels.

- If the egg is fertilized, the baby's placenta will eventually take over the ovary's job and will produce a huge amount (300 times normal) of progesterone during the pregnancy. (The strong estrogen, E2, on the other hand, only increases 100 times normal during pregnancy.)

- All that **estrogen makes you retain fat** and reduces muscle mass to make sure you can stay in the "nest" and continue to feed your fetus off your body fat stores even if food is scarce.

- If there is **no pregnancy**, both **estrogen and progesterone fall** and the uterine lining is discarded (**you get your period**).

It's important to understand that, outside of pregnancy, *your only meaningful source of progesterone comes from your ovaries after each month's ovulation.*

If you don't ovulate in a given month, *you do not make enough progesterone* to balance the estrogen your body continues to make.

WHEN YOU DON'T OVULATE

Notice how different the month's chart (below) looks when you *don't* ovulate.

You continue to make a lot of estrogen, building up that uterine lining, clotting blood, storing fat and reducing muscle mass, while growing milk-secreting cells in the breast in preparation for a pregnancy, but *there is no progesterone in the second half of the month to put the brakes on* all that activity.

*Progesterone is **vitally** important to balance the effects of estrogen, especially to slow the rate of cell division and to normalize clotting.*

WHY YOU MIGHT NOT OVULATE

Among the most common reasons for failure to ovulate are:
- Pregnancy
- Polycystic ovary syndrome (PCOS)
- Hormone imbalance (too much prolactin, too little thyroxine)
- Low body weight
- Obesity, insulin resistance

- Excessive exercise/training
- Menopause
- Chronic illness
- Drugs (especially anti-inflammatories, chemo, cocaine)

A Month with NO Ovulation

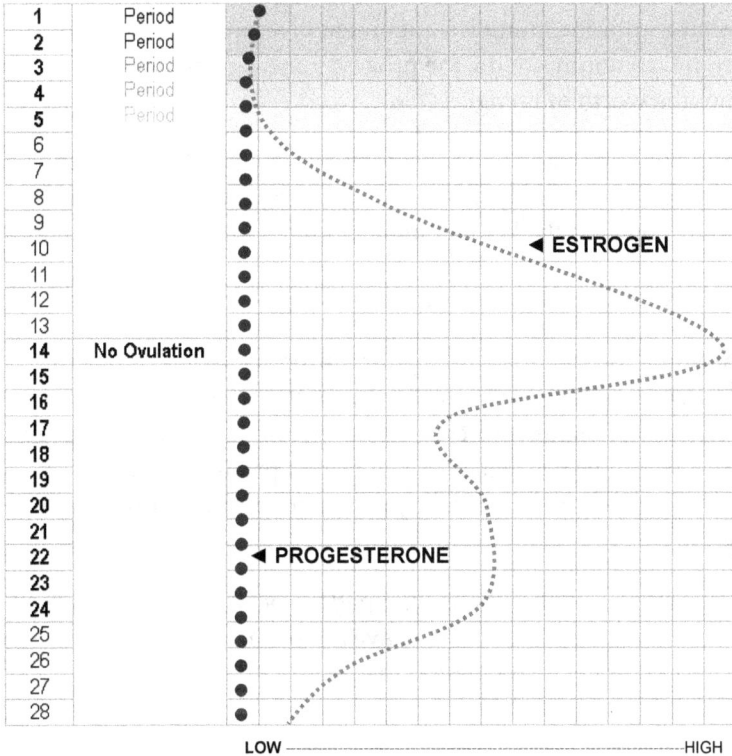

1	Period	
2	Period	
3	Period	
4	Period	
5	Period	
6		
7		
8		
9		
10		◀ ESTROGEN
11		
12		
13		
14	No Ovulation	
15		
16		
17		
18		
19		
20		
21		
22		◀ PROGESTERONE
23		
24		
25		
26		
27		
28		

LOW ———————————————————————————— HIGH

REMEMBER: The longer your body is exposed to estrogen without a sufficient amount of progesterone, the more likely you are to develop cancers of the uterus, cervix, ovaries or breasts.

SYMPTOMS OF FAILURE TO OVULATE & MAKE PROGESTERONE

You probably already know that if you don't ovulate you can't get pregnant.

What you may *not* know is that when you don't ovulate in a given month, your next period may be *lighter*. The reason is that, without progesterone to soften the uterine lining, the lining may not discard completely during your period.

For the same reasons, you may have an *unusually heavy* period the following month when you *do* ovulate, because the current month's uterine lining is built on top of whatever was left over from last month's. Now the progesterone is softening two-months worth of lining.

And because estrogen has been ruling your body ("estrogen dominance") for at least a month and a half, the blood in that lining could be thicker and more clotted than in a normal month.

CHANGES AT MENOPAUSE

As you approach the end of your reproductive years (the time known as "perimenopause," or the period *around* menopause), more and more of your cycles fly by without producing an egg. And as you've learned, when you don't produce a mature egg (ovulate), you don't produce progesterone, and estrogen runs amok.

The first sign of this change is a pattern of wildly erratic cycles. For several months you may have almost no periods, or you may have one really heavy period that seems to last forever.

That happens because, without progesterone during those non-ovulatory months, your body has been unable to completely flush out the old uterine lining. And as the months continue without progesterone, the lining gets thicker and thicker, because estrogen is still doing its job.

Remember that even though you may be producing less estrogen as you get older, you still have considerably more of it than progesterone when you don't ovulate.

SYMPTOMS OF MENOPAUSE OR PERIMENOPAUSE

The hormone losses and imbalances that occur around and after menopause can produce a number of symptoms, including:

Hot flashes	Breast/nipple tenderness
Night Sweats	Decreased nipple sensitivity
Heart palpitations	Reduced/increased sex drive
Irregular/skipped periods	Leaking urine/incontinence
Heavy/long periods	Mood swings/irritability
Chronic fatigue	Depression/anxiety
Random pains/fibromyalgia	Brain fog/poor memory
Dry, itchy/crawly skin	Ovarian cysts
Vaginal dryness	Endometriosis
Weight gain	Fibroids
Carb/sugar cravings	Fluid retention/bloating
Hair loss/thinning/excess hair	New/worsening allergies
Headaches	Autoimmune diseases
Infertility/miscarriage	Muscle wasting
Insomnia	Osteoporosis
High cholesterol	Dry eyes, dry mouth
Senses less acute (esp. smell)	Indigestion, heartburn
Loss of creativity, passions	Poor coordination
Red neck with white center	Acne

While several of these can occur during reproductive years for any number of reasons that may or may not be connected with hormones, the presence of a large number of these symptoms may suggest that you are approaching the menopausal transition.

WHAT EXACTLY HAPPENS AT MENOPAUSE?

When you reach menopause, you are no longer ovulating and, therefore, your ovaries are not making progesterone.

Menopause can occur naturally, or can be brought on abruptly by surgical removal of the ovaries (oophorectomy) and sometimes by hysterectomy (see "Hysterectomy and Your Hormones," below).

In the natural winding down of your reproductive system, several significant events occur:

➤ **Estrogen and testosterone production declines.**

- Your ovaries may continue to produce smaller and smaller amounts of estrogen and testosterone as the brain realizes you're not ovulating anymore.

- But your adrenal glands continue to make testosterone, a small amount of estrogen and a tiny amount of progesterone.

- Your body fat also continues to convert a certain amount of your testosterone and other hormones into estrogen.

➤ **Progesterone production drops dramatically.**

- You have no meaningful backup sources of progesterone, so when the ovaries shut down, your progesterone levels drop like a rock and stay there.

➤ **Feedback hormones in the brain start yelling.**

- When the brain detects low hormone levels in the ovaries, it starts "yelling"—increasing the amount of ovulation-stimulating hormones like FSH.

- Normally FSH would only yell (or surge) at ovulation time. In response, the body would boost estrogen output to mature the egg and get it out of the follicle and on its way. Then FSH levels would drop again.

- But when there is no response to the brain's demand for more estrogen, the FSH remains high, continuing to yell.

After Menopause

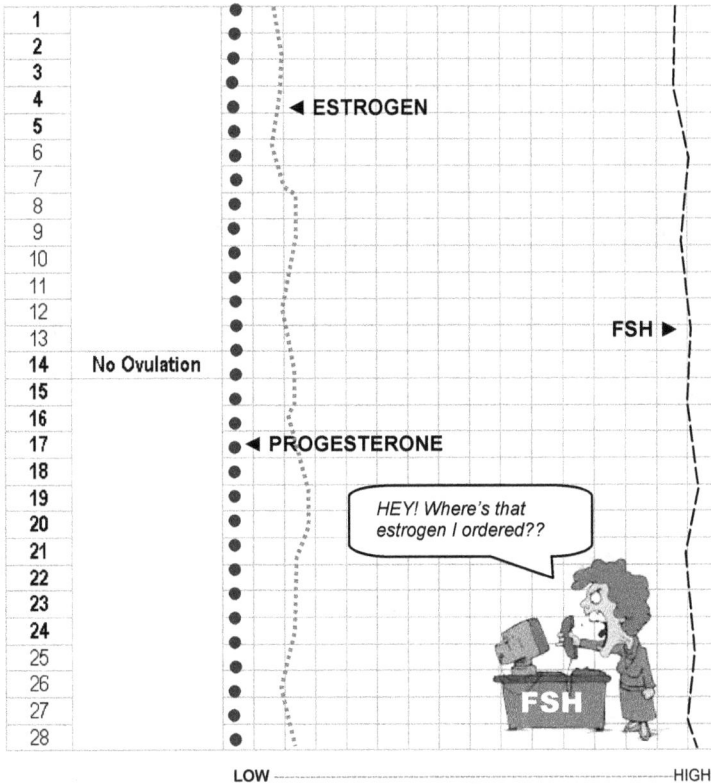

- That's when you start having hot flashes and other dramatic symptoms of estrogen withdrawal.

- For many women, the brain eventually realizes the estrogen is not coming and those initial symptoms subside.

How is Menopause Diagnosed?

In the past, **menopause** was diagnosed when a woman had gone **without a period for 12 consecutive months**.

But these days, it's a little harder to tell, especially with women using hormonal birth control methods.

In fact, if you use contraceptive hormones, you may not know when your ovaries shut down, because the fake estrogen and progesterone in the contraceptives will continue to produce periods on a regular basis.

Fortunately, today's medical science is able to detect a more precise state of natural menopause ("chemical or hormonal menopause"), at least in women who are not taking hormones.

Chemical/hormonal menopause is reached when:

- Your **FSH** is continuously *above* **25 mIU/mL** *and...*

- Your **estradiol** estrogen level (E2) is *below* **50 pg/mL**

KEY MENOPAUSE INDICATORS

FSH continuously above 25 mIU/mL

FSH HIGH

E2 LOW

Estradiol (E2) below 50 pg/mL

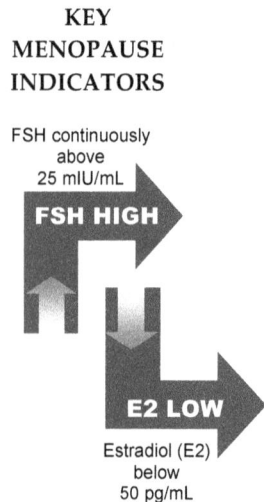

In fact, you can get over-the-counter, dipstick-type FSH tests. Like pregnancy tests, they require you to test your morning's urine and then they display a positive reading if your FSH is above 25 mIU/mL. *(See Urine Tests in Chapter 12.)*

FSH *alone* cannot tell you whether you've quit ovulating permanently, but it can provide a clue that it may be time to consult your doctor.

The combination of consistently high FSH and low E2 estrogen provides a sure sign of hormonal menopause, even if you are still getting periods.

WHEN DOES MENOPAUSE OCCUR?

Nature designed our bodies to be fertile only when we are fat enough to sustain a pregnancy to term. So it's not unusual for rail-thin models, athletes or anorexics to stop ovulating for months at a time. Their periods may become very light or stop completely. But that's not menopause.

When these women get back to a relatively normal weight, their periods—and their fertility—will likely return.

Menopause, on the other hand is permanent. Your ovaries have used up their eggs and there's no coming back.

- **Most women (70%) reach menopause between the ages of 48 and 55.** However, for 5% of us it happens even later.

- What may surprise you is that about **one in four of us (25%) will enter menopause** *before* **the age of 47.**

- And **35 to 58 is** considered the **"typical" age range for natural menopause** to occur.

You read that correctly: It is considered *typical* for women as young as 35 to be entering menopause!

No matter what your age when you hit menopause (or *it* hits *you*), you don't have to accept all the baggage that goes with it. That's why we're here: to help you stay young even after Mother Nature decides to retire.

HYSTERECTOMY AND YOUR HORMONES

Hysterectomy, when it includes removal of the ovaries, creates an instantaneous state of menopause, no matter how young the woman.

Belief once was that by leaving a woman's ovaries intact and only removing her uterus in a hysterectomy, doctors could at least keep the woman's hormone factories squirting out hormones.

What medical science has since discovered is that **in as many as 50% of cases, a woman's ovaries shut down or reduce function within three years of her hysterectomy**. This may be the result of damage to important nerves and blood supplies to the ovaries. If so, more advanced surgical techniques may improve this situation.

In any case, if you are thinking of having a hysterectomy for non-life-threatening reasons (heavy periods, birth control) and assume that if you keep your ovaries you will maintain youthful levels of sex hormones, you might want to reconsider.

At least discuss this issue with your surgeon to determine what steps can be taken to preserve your ovarian function after surgery.

HOW FAR DO YOUR SEX HORMONES DROP?

After menopause, your three main sex hormones will have dropped significantly to new levels. In the process you lose approximately:

- 50% of your testosterone

- 65% of your estrogen *(depending upon how much fat you have and how much testosterone you have that is converting into estrogen)*

- 90% of your progesterone

One of the most disturbing aspects of this transition is the *uneven* drop in hormone levels.

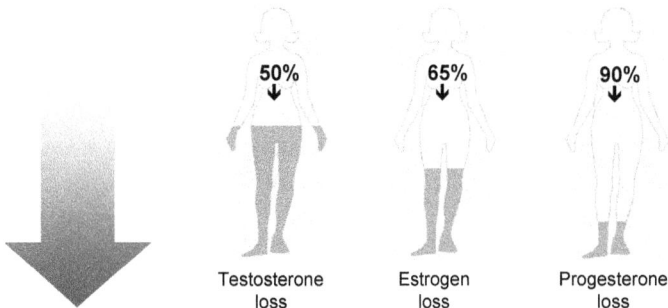

50% ↓	65% ↓	90% ↓
Testosterone loss	Estrogen loss	Progesterone loss

All of our hormones are designed to operate in specific proportions relative to one other. When levels begin to drop at different rates, those critical proportions are thrown off, and the systems, processes and organs that depend on those balanced hormones can suffer significantly.

Consider this: Your stomach contains hydrochloric acid (HCL), which is strong enough to eat through concrete. But it doesn't eat through your stomach because the stomach has a protective lining of mucus.

Now imagine what would happen if, as you got older, both your acid and mucus levels dropped. You'd be fine if they dropped evenly. But if the mucus dropped far more than the acid, you'd be full of ulcers. And if the acid dropped more than the mucus, your food would never digest, it would sit in your stomach and rot. (This actually happens to some extent as we age.)

So, while it is important to boost hormones that are low, it is far more important to maintain proper proportions of hormones, whether they are left low or are supplemented.

ESTROGEN DOMINANCE

As mentioned earlier, when your body doesn't make enough progesterone, estrogen "rules" your body. Some researchers now believe that when estrogen is allowed to rule too long it can lead to cancers that may not show up until many years later.

When your body is in a state of **"estrogen dominance,"** it has too little counterbalancing progesterone to curb estrogen's desire to stimulate cell growth (cell division) and other functions.

While this cell division/growth helps your body prepare for conception and for gestating and then nursing a baby, **nature never intended for estrogen to operate without the proper** *opposing* **forces**.

Back in the 1970s, when horse estrogen (Premarin) was all the rage for making women feel young again after menopause, doctors began to notice that a lot of women who had not had hysterectomies were developing **uterine (endometrial) cancer.**

When the researchers looked at younger women's hormones (since they typically didn't get that type of cancer) they noticed that estrogen was always balanced by a much larger amount of progesterone.

So the drug company created a synthetic version of progesterone (since real /bio-identical progesterone can't be patented) and added it to the horse estrogen to be taken by women who still had a uterus. And that reduced the rate of endometrial cancer dramatically.

What these researchers didn't consider was that **unopposed estrogen was just as damaging in other organs, like the ovaries and breasts, as it was in the uterus.** And they didn't realize that *all* women needed progesterone.

The scientists could make a nice neat connection between taking horse estrogen alone and uterine cancer. But with diseases like breast cancer, however, the connection was much harder to see because in many cases the *effect* didn't occur for years or even decades after the *cause*.

But now many researchers have. And from that connection, they have developed the **"estrogen window hypothesis."**

THE "ESTROGEN WINDOW" HYPOTHESIS

This hypothesis proposes that **diseases like breast cancer**—which seem to be more prevalent among postmenopausal women—**may actually be triggered during that period around 5-10 years** *before* **menopause** *when a woman is still making lots of estrogen, but is not producing enough progesterone to counteract the estrogen effects.*

As we've discussed earlier, estrogen typically *does not* cause cancer, not even when it's unopposed by progesterone.

But what it *does* is increase the frenzy of cell division and cell growth in various organs, especially the uterus, ovary and breasts. And when that happens it becomes harder for your immune system to catch all the mutant cells that randomly appear in any given division cycle and flush them out of your body.

If you also happen to be under a lot of stress, are sleeping poorly, aren't getting enough vitamin D3, or are simply growing older, your immune system won't be operating at its peak and will find it harder still to stay ahead of all the random mutants popping up.

The other key piece of this puzzle is that a given breast tumor may take up to 7-10 years to grow from the first little cluster of mutants into a detectable mass.

That's why researchers missed the connection between unopposed estrogen and breast cancer for so long.

Progressive healthcare practitioners today know that it can be vitally important to **supplement** a woman's **progesterone** as soon as she begins having multiple non-ovulatory cycles in order to *prevent* the conditions that can lead to later diagnoses of *breast and other estrogen-related cancers*.

HORMONE-RELATED CANCERS

Although this is a book for women, as long as we're discussing hormone-related cancers that can be easily prevented, I would like to briefly mention the similar cases of prostate and breast cancers in men.

Men can suffer from estrogen dominance too, but in men it relates more to the balance between estrogen and the opposing forces of testosterone, primarily, and progesterone. Too little testosterone—or too little testosterone relative to the level of estrogen—can lead to breast and prostate cancer in men.

In fact, numerous studies (including the 2004 Baltimore Longitudinal Study of Aging, and 2006 USC studies) are now showing that *men with the lowest levels of testosterone have the highest risk of prostate cancer*.

Many doctors are now supplementing testosterone in men to prevent diseases like prostate cancer, breast cancer and even Alzheimer's and Parkinson's disease.

Although no testosterone studies have been conducted on women, studies indicate a similar connection between low estrogen and an increased risk of Alzheimer's. Further research may eventually tell us more about the role of testosterone and other hormones in various disease processes.

THE 2/16 RATIO

The strong estrogens your body makes (or the bio-identicals that you supplement) can break down in two main ways: either into the 2 version or the 16 version. (Technically, these metabolites, or waste products of estrogen, have long chemical names, but all you have to remember is the 2 and 16.)

As it turns out, the 16 version stimulates a lot of cell division and is far more strongly associated with hormone-related cancers than the 2 version.

But you can help encourage your body to break down your estrogen into the more beneficial 2 version by eating plenty of "cruciferous" vegetables like broccoli, cauliflower, cabbage, and Brussels sprouts. (And don't worry if you can't stand to eat any of these; you can still get their nutrients in supplement form.)

You can actually test your 2/16 ratio to find out how well you are encouraging the favorable conversion of your estrogens, or to monitor the impact of your dietary changes on the 2/16 ratio.

A DAY IN THE LIFE OF YOUR HORMONES

Have you ever wondered how your hormones ebb and flow throughout the day to keep your body running, and then resting, all in the right sequences? Well, here's a glimpse into the secret life of your hormones...

NIGHT

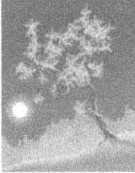

Overnight, your sequences of **restorative REM sleep** help you perform needed repairs and data processing. And *in the darkness*, your pineal gland shuts off **cortisol** and produces **melatonin**, which helps you sleep...and **lowers** your production of **estrogen** to keep it under control and to reduce your risk of estrogen-sensitive cancers. If you already have **low estrogen**, this surge of estrogen-suppressing **melatonin** may bring on a passing heat wave or even a night sweat around 3:00 am. In the absence of food to process, your liver produces **glycogen** to break down the **glucose (blood sugar)** stored in your cells for fuel.

DAWN

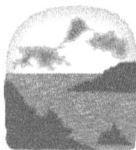

The faint light coming through your window tells your **pineal** gland that it's time to stop making **melatonin** so you can begin to wake up. Your **adrenal** glands pump out your highest regular **cortisol** dose of the day to perk you up, plus a little dose of **adrenalin/epinephrine** that quickens your pulse and narrows blood vessels (increases blood pressure) to get you out of bed and on your feet.

BREAKFAST

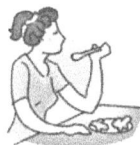

Your **stomach** produces the hormone **ghrelin,** which makes you feel hungry after the long night's fast. And it produces **histamine**, which in turn triggers the release of **gastric acid (HCL)** and enzymes to help break down your food. As you eat, the carbohydrates in your breakfast break down into **glucose** (blood sugar). This tells your **pancreas** to produce **insulin,** which moves that glucose into the cells of your organs and muscles to store for fuel. The **gallbladder** releases **bile** to break down proteins so your body can use them to build tissues. **Hormones** in your gastro-intestinal **(GI) tract** increase the movement in your gut and continue breaking down your food so its nutrients can be absorbed into your bloodstream.

EXERCISE

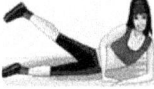

As you work out, your body burns the **glucose** (sugar) stored in your muscles. If you run or exercise hard enough, your **pituitary** will start making **endorphins**, those feel-good chemicals. They also help dampen pains, just like morphine. The hormone **leptin** in the fat you're burning increases your metabolism and reduces your appetite (if everything else is working properly). Your **heart** secretes a **peptide** which tells the **kidneys** to produce urine. Now you get thirsty and your body may crave water and perhaps electrolytes like salt and potassium.

SUNSHINE

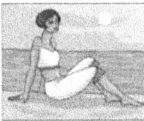

On a nice sunny day, you might get outside to the beach or go for a walk. If you sweat and expose plenty of skin for at least 10-20 minutes (depending on your age and skin color), your **skin** produces as much as 10,000 to 20,000 IUs of immune-turbocharging **vitamin D** before you have to cover up or put on sunscreen for protection. If a cool breeze comes in while you're wet in your swimsuit, you may start to shiver, which indicates that your **thyroid** has released more of its hormones to step up your metabolism to keep you warm.

DAYTIME

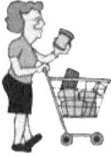

As you go about your daily tasks, your **pituitary** tells the **thyroid** to make **hormones** that regulate your metabolism and keep your body temperature where it should be. It also tells your **ovaries** and **adrenals** to produce **estrogen** and **testosterone** to maintain sexual processes and to support your brain, bones, muscles and mood. And **growth hormone** from the **pituitary** keeps your body growing and/or renewing according to nature's blueprint. If your blood calcium drops too low or your pH is too acidic, your **parathyroid gland** secretes a **parathyroid hormone** that steals calcium from **bones** and **muscles** to neutralize the acid.

STRESS

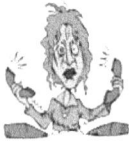

As you face stressful situations, your **adrenals** squirt out extra doses of **cortisol** to mobilize emergency energy from your muscles and organs. The more stressful your life, the more your adrenal glands are taxed, until they eventually can burn out and become unable to produce even normal levels of cortisol. If your **estrogen** levels are already low or fluctuating wildly, you may experience heart palpitations or an occasional hot flash.

EXTREME
STRESS

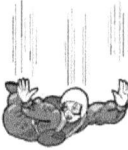

If you experience fear or shock or any kind of extreme stress (even desired shocks, like a marriage proposal or pregnancy news, or performing daredevil stunts) during the day, your **adrenal** glands will also pump out the "fight-or-flight" hormone **adrenalin** (**epinephrine**). This makes your heart race, increases blood pressure, and generally prepares your body to do battle or outrun danger.

MEALS,
SNACKS

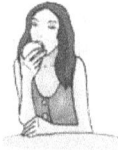

If you make a point to eat small, healthy meals and snacks about every three hours during the day—including some protein and complex carbs—your **pancreas** will have no trouble keeping your **insulin** and **glucose/blood sugar** levels stable. A calcium-rich snack replaces any calcium your **parathyroid hormone** robbed earlier from your **bones** and **muscles** to stabilize blood calcium and pH, and tells the **parathyroid gland** to produce **calcitonin** (made from **vitamin D**) to put the calcium back.

OVULATION

If you are still fertile, and it's the middle of the menstrual month, your **pituitary** shoots out a burst of **FSH**, telling your **ovaries** to raise **estrogen** to its monthly peak, forcing the matured egg out of the ovary. In the empty ovarian **follicle**, the **ovary** now produces **progesterone** that softens both the uterine lining and your mood for the next two weeks, and helps build healthy brain, bone and muscle, while balancing the effects of your estrogen.

EVENING

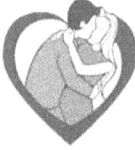

As you think about that special person in your life, your **ovaries** and **adrenals** secrete **testosterone** to make you feel sexy and to have sexual fantasies. Thinking about him, or finally seeing him may cause your **adrenals** to squirt out **adrenaline/epinephrine**, giving your heart that pitterpatter feeling. During sex, your **pituitary** produces those lovely **endorphins** that make you feel so good. To help you climax, the **pituitary** releases **oxytocin**—the same hormone that produces the contractions of childbirth and causes breast milk to "let down" or flow. **Oxytocin** promotes bonding emotions, and with its cousin, **prolactin** (from the **pituitary** and the **uterus**), the two make you feel satisfied and snuggly in the afterglow of love.

NIGHT

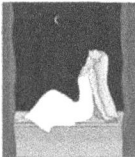

By the end of the day, your supplies of **cortisol** are getting low. You may have had a surge or two during the day giving you a little boost, but they are falling now. You may still have some **adrenalin** circulating after some stresses or excitement that needs to be burned off with some light exercise. If you have a late snack, it's best to get one with protein so its **tryptophan** can break down into the mood-leveling **serotonin**. And finally, as you dim and then turn off the lights, your **pineal** gland starts to produce **melatonin** and you drift off to sleep.

As you can see, your hormones are critical for nearly everything your body does. And minimizing the stress (and its hormones) in your life may be the number one secret to remaining youthful.

15 | Nutritional/Digestive Processes

Your healthy nutritional processes depend upon both the substances you put into your body (food, drink, supplements) and the digestive system that makes those substances suitable for use by your body.

Organs and Glands

The key organs/glands that serve the nutritional and digestive processes are:

- Mouth and salivary glands
- Esophagus
- Stomach
- Gallbladder
- Small intestine
- Large intestine (colon)

The diagram below shows you generally where these organs are located and how they are connected.

The digestive system needs the right substances in order to do its job. Some of the most important are:

- **Saliva** (breaks down food and makes swallowing easier)
- **Histamine** (stimulates gastric/stomach acid)
- **Stomach acid/HCL** (kills food bacteria and parasites)
- **Mucus** (protects the stomach from its acid)
- **Digestive enzymes: pepsin, bile, etc**. (process food further)
- **Friendly gut bacteria** (protect intestinal lining)
- **Serotonin** (increases appetite, regulates intestinal movements)

Organs of the Nutritional/Digestive System

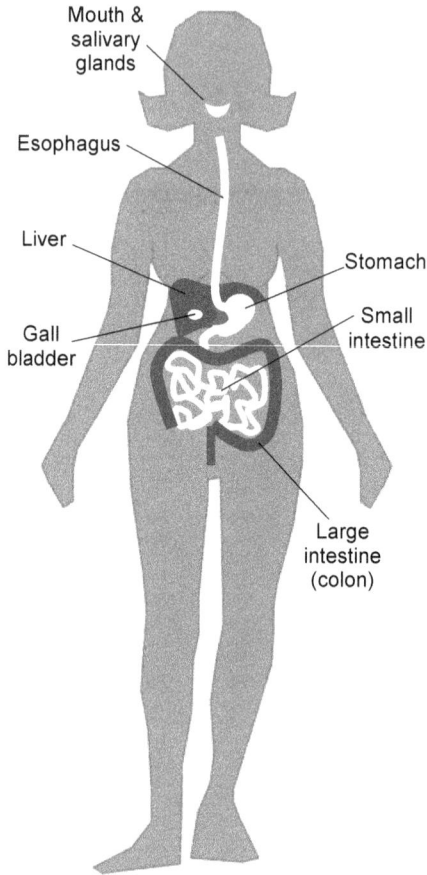

As you can guess from the roles each of these elements play, a decrease in the level of one or more of them—or an imbalance between them—can wreak havoc with your health.

In fact, it is said that 75% of your immune system resides in your gut!

Like every other process in your body, the digestive/nutritional processes depend on other systems in order to do their jobs. Without hormones, or the nerves that help your body communicate, or the ability to remove toxins, you could not reap the benefit of the foods you consume.

The Digestion Process

The first stop in the process of obtaining nutrients from food is your mouth where saliva and chewing begin to break down what you eat into manageable chunks.

One of the best things you can do for your gut is to chew your food thoroughly before swallowing.

The food goes down the esophagus and is pushed downward by one-way muscles and valves. If they are weak or damaged, you may experience acid reflux or heartburn.

In the stomach, histamine releases gastric acid (HCL) and other substances (especially the enzyme *pepsin*), which further reduce the components of your meal and begin to make their nutrients accessible for absorption.

But it's in the small intestine where the real work begins, where the broken-down bits slowly move through and dissolve even more in the presence of bile and enzymes from the pancreas, gallbladder and liver, passing nutrients into your bloodstream.

And finally, in the colon (large intestine), the unusable waste products, fiber, and toxins are pushed on their way toward the exit where they are eliminated in a bowel movement.

The Stomach Acid/Heartburn Paradox

One of the most common digestive complaints—especially in older women—is heartburn (acid reflux/GERD or indigestion). And the most common solutions include antacids or acid-reducing medications.

Occasionally, the problem truly is related to excess stomach acid. But here's the secret: In many cases, the problem isn't *too much* stomach acid, but *too little!* It seems backwards, but once you think about it, it'll make perfect sense.

The hydrochloric acid (HCL) your stomach produces is designed to kill bacteria and parasites, promote the absorption of vitamin B-12, and jump-start the process of breaking down food in your stomach.

But as you get older, you make less HCL. With too little HCL, your food sits in your stomach longer, *rotting* instead of quickly breaking down into smaller bits your intestines can handle. That bacterial decay process can cause gas (burping) and that feeling of food coming back up into your throat.

Too little HCL can allow bad bacteria to flourish in your gut, can cause recurrent yeast infections, and may trigger inflammation that can damage the cardiovascular system and cause "leaky gut syndrome," which can lead to autoimmune conditions.

And when you don't break down food properly, a whole host of problems can arise—from hair loss (too little accessible protein), to macular degeneration of your eyes, and overall reduced or out-of-control immune function.

The solution then is simple: take an HCL pill at the beginning of each meal to help accelerate the breakdown process in your stomach. The HCL supplement may include pepsin, an enzyme that also aids digestion.

Just remember that not everyone's heartburn is caused by too little HCL.

TESTING FOR LOW HCL

A simple test is to drink a small amount (1/4 teaspoon in water) of baking soda first thing in the morning. If you have not burped within a few minutes, you may not be making enough HCL.

A more definitive test for low HCL involves measuring the amount of undigested protein in the stool.

Another way to test is to take an HCL pill at the start of a meal. If you truly have too much acid in your stomach, you will begin to experience symptoms of heartburn/acid reflux. If that occurs, you can take a teaspoon of baking soda in water (or an antacid) to quickly neutralize the acid. On the other hand, if you get no reaction, or if your heartburn improves upon taking the HCL, you can probably benefit from taking HCL regularly with meals.

Friendly Gut Bacteria

As we've mentioned, the gut is an important fortress in your body's immune system. And the friendly bacteria that live there are critical to keeping toxins from passing through the walls of the intestines and into your bloodstream.

Even E. coli — the bug that seems to cause so much trouble when it shows up where it doesn't belong (in food or in your bladder) — is essential for helping your gut finish the digestion process, getting the last drop of nutrients from your food.

So a part of your optimal wellness plan has to include maintaining those bacteria at their normal levels.

Illness and antibiotics are among the common causes of reduced gut bacteria. And probiotics (pills or foods like yogurt that contain these beneficial bacteria) provide a solution.

Case of the Missing Nutrients

Most nutritionists will tell you that whole food is the best source of nutrients. And that would be true if those foods were grown naturally, without pesticides, in nutrient-rich soil and delivered within a short time of harvesting.

Unfortunately, most foods today are gown in depleted soil, and may be processed—or even bred—for long shelf-life. That means the apples you bought yesterday may have been picked two years ago, then coated in wax and stored in a warehouse before being shipped to your grocery store.

FRESH VS. FROZEN

Logically, it would seem that vegetables, meats and fish from the fresh section of the store would be more healthful. But sometimes the frozen products are a better choice. Those "fresh" products may have been preserved or frozen and stored then thawed, losing much of their nutrients along the way.

Frozen products, on the other hand, are typically flash frozen shortly after harvesting or processing, and are kept frozen throughout their shelf lives. Depending on how long they've been stored, these products may have more nutritional value than so-called fresh items.

NUTRITIONAL SUPPLEMENTS

The fact is that to get all the nutrients you need, you may have to depend on supplements.

A micronutrients test may be the best way to find out which nutrients you are missing.

Food Sensitivities/Allergies

For some, food allergies or sensitivities can cause a whole range of dysfunctions. They can include:

- Rashes and skin irritations/bumps
- Rheumatoid arthritis
- Headaches
- Bowel irregularities

The traditional allergy scratch tests can identify some of these foods. But other substances may not react in your system for hours or days. Because of the delay, you may not make the connection between the reaction and a cause that may have occurred days before.

That's why it may be helpful to conduct tests for food sensitivities using an IgG blood test.

THE ELIMINATION DIET

The simplest test is the elimination diet. You remove all but the most harmless foods from your diet, then wait a few days until your symptoms subside. Then you start adding foods back in, one at a time, every few days. If your bothersome symptoms return, you remove the most recent substance from your diet, wait till symptoms fade, then add something new.

This process can take a long time, but it is effective in identifying foods you are sensitive to so you can avoid them.

FOOD ALLERGY TESTING

The IgG blood test, on the other hand, can help diagnose food sensitivities, but do it much faster.

LEAKY GUT SYNDROME

A healthy mucosal lining in the gut keeps out about 98% of antigens (substances the immune system recognizes as invaders) that might otherwise penetrate the lining of the gut and get into your bloodstream.

Troublesome antigens can include components of foods as well as parasites and yeasts.

When the mucosal lining of the gut breaks down (with age or due to various assaults on your digestive system, including drugs or stress), more antigens are able to penetrate or leak through the barrier.

When you have a "leaky gut," the levels of various antigens rise throughout your body, which triggers your immune system to go on the attack to stop and eliminate these invaders.

This, in turn, creates inflammation, which can lead to conditions such as arthritis, irritable bowel syndrome, and even heart disease and cancer.

16| Nervous System & Communication Processes

We don't need a diagram to show you that virtually every part of your body is connected to the brain through a vast network of nerves.

The key parts of the nervous system are:

- Brain
- Spinal cord
- Peripheral nerves
- Myelin sheath

The **spinal column** carries information to and from the **brain**. And the **peripheral nerves** that branch off from it **provide two-way communication between individual systems and the brain**.

As you've already learned, the brain contains glands that produce chemicals that make your various processes work properly. You've seen how one gland may secrete a chemical that, in turn, makes another gland produce (or stop producing) its own chemicals.

But the nervous system is also involved in this process, **communicating signals from one organ to another**, to tell a certain organ to produce a chemical, or to release a chemical that *counteracts* the effect of another one.

Your brain and your nervous system tell your body to start releasing insulin to process that chocolate-covered strawberry you've just treated yourself to while reading this book. And it happens automatically. You don't have to think about it.

The nervous system (along with the chemicals released by the endocrine/hormonal system) tells the muscles in your digestive tract to start squeezing to process that food. And it keeps the squeezing process (peristalsis) *synchronized* so that the food moves forward…from the stomach…to the small intestine…to the large intestine (colon)…and finally out into the toilet.

In a similar fashion, the nervous system is essential to the operation of every other organ and system in your body. That's why it's important to maintain the integrity of the nervous system and keep the channels of communication open.

Myelin: the Nervous System's Protection

The **myelin sheath** is like the outer coating on an electrical extension cord. It protects the nerves (and the brain) from damage and from short circuiting. If that sheath is worn or if it is not as thick as it should be, the nerves inside may be easily damaged.

Curiously, as Dr. John Lee and others note, the **cells that maintain this myelin sheath contain receptors for the hormone progesterone**. This may be among the biggest clues of all that the sex hormones are not just for reproduction.

The presence of these receptors tells us that your brain and nervous system depend upon the presence of progesterone in order to maintain their protective coating. And if progesterone levels are allowed to drop without supplementation (either during non-ovulatory months of your cycle or after menopause), you could experience disruptions in any number of other systems as a result of lost or garbled communications.

Nervous System Dysfunction

If a nerve is constricted or pinched by a bone, disc or scar tissue, it can cut off or reduce the transmission of information in the same way pinching a garden hose can reduce or stop the flow of water. Exactly where the nerve is pinched will determine which organs or systems are affected.

Chiropractic treatment may be the best first step in relieving misalignments that impair the flow of information throughout your body's nervous system. If you have a serious structural dysfunction, you may even need surgery

If you have a deficiency in the myelin sheath, it can create a kind of short circuit that keeps signals from getting to their intended destinations or may cause signals to be sent to the wrong destinations.

Because progesterone plays an important role in maintaining that myelin sheath, it follows that low progesterone levels can, over time, increase your susceptibility to nerve dysfunction. It may even cause random pains for no apparent reason or cause numbness in affected parts of your body. Some even suspect that progesterone deficiency may be a contributor to multiple sclerosis and fibromyalgia in some patients.

FIBROMYALGIA & CHRONIC FATIGUE

These conditions often plague many post-menopausal women.

FIBROMYALGIA

Fibromyalgia sufferers report pain and tenderness in a variety of joints, muscles, tendons and other soft tissues throughout the body, though no conventional medical tests can find a specific cause for those pains, and the diagnosis is often controversial.

Its other symptoms are strikingly similar to those of low or imbalanced sex hormones, including fatigue, sleep disturbances, brain fog, and depression/anxiety.

Because progesterone is needed for proper nerve protection, it seems reasonable that a progesterone deficiency—and possibly deficiencies in the myelin sheath—could be responsible for the apparent misfiring of the nervous system in fibromyalgia.

Not surprisingly (at least to me), one of the most effective treatments for fibromyalgia involves supplementing and balancing the sex hormones (especially progesterone), along with high doses of intravenous (IV) vitamins and nutrients.

Chronic Fatigue Syndrome

Chronic fatigue is another controversial condition that is often ignored or ascribed to other causes. And it frequently goes hand-in-hand with fibromyalgia.

Chronic fatigue is debilitating fatigue that persists for more than 24 hours, and it may sometimes continue for years. It can also be accompanied by aches (myalgias) and other symptoms, including those common to low or imbalanced sex hormones. Fortunately, the same treatments (hormones and nutrients) used for fibromyalgia may resolve chronic fatigue as well.

SUBLUXATIONS AND SPINAL MISALIGNMENTS

Because the spine is the main highway of your nervous system, any misalignments or kinks in that highway can lead to faulty or missing communications farther out in the network. A kink in the neck could worsen your allergies while another kink farther down could produce bladder issues.

Chiropractic therapy helps identify misalignments (subluxations) and correct them by manipulating the connections between vertebrae and realigning them.

17 | Purification Processes: Immune & Detoxification Systems

The process of rejecting invaders and detoxifying your body starts with identifying toxins and attacking, disabling or sequestering them. Then your system must release the toxins from your tissues, and finally flush them out of your body.

Organs and Glands

To perform their functions, these systems rely on a number of organs and mechanisms, including:

- **Salivary glands** / saliva (breaks down food)

- **Bone marrow** / white blood cells, etc. (immune system)

- **Sweat glands** / sweat (releases fat-soluble toxins through the skin)

- **Lymph glands** / lymphatic fluid (manufacture white cells, fight off infection and filter out toxins and other harmful invaders)

- **Liver** (filters out toxins and prepares them for removal)

- **Kidneys** / urine (filters toxins and removes via urination)

- **Colon** / stool (processes and removes toxins via bowel movement)

Organs of the Immune & Detoxification Systems

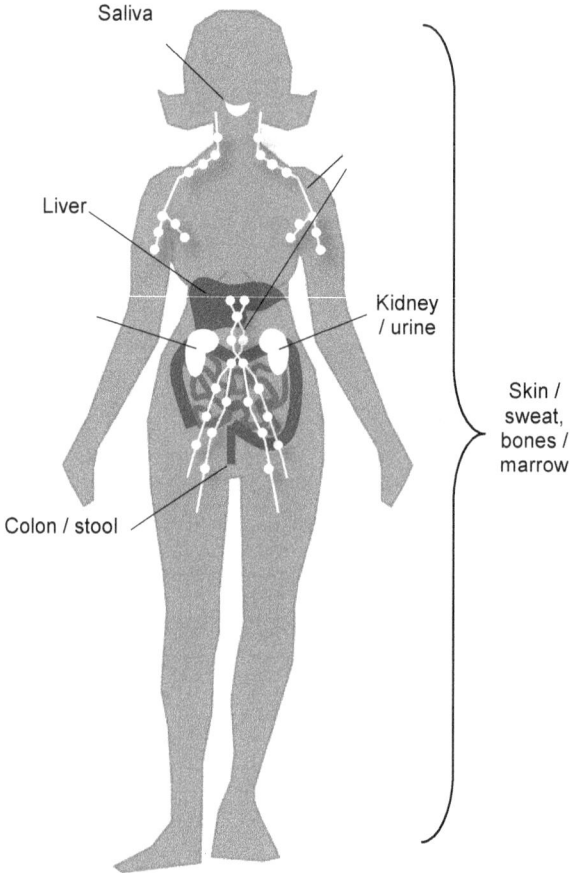

What this diagram can't show is the vast **lymphatic network** that branches like blood vessels from head to toe throughout the body, with "**nodes**" at various intersections to collect/filter out harmful substances.

Immune Response

Your body's first step in protecting your health is to **recognize harmful agents and disable them**. That's primarily the job of your immune system.

If you get a splinter in your finger, for example, your immune system recognizes it as an invader and triggers inflammation in the skin surrounding it.

This process ideally will push the invader out. But if the splinter won't come out, the immune and detoxification systems will start to eat away at it in an effort to process it out of your body that way.

And if the splinter turns out to be too deeply embedded in your skin, or is made of some hard-to-decompose substance, the immune system will simply build a wall around it, often made of calcium, until that wall encapsulates the invader in a shell that resembles concrete so that it cannot interfere with your health.

In a similar manner, your healthy immune system raises a flag whenever it sees an invader of any kind, then sends its armies to attack and disable it one way or another, often passing the remains on to your detoxification centers for elimination.

Remember that the majority of your immune system (75%) resides in your gut.

Your healthy immune system may be the single most important weapon in the battle for long-term wellness, youthfulness and overall longevity.

That's why so many of the solutions you'll find in this book focus on supporting and boosting your immune system.

INFLAMMATION, FEVER, PAIN

When your body is attacked by anything it recognizes as alien, your immune system mounts a defense. That defense releases hormone-like substances called *eicosanoids*.

These eicosanoids (prostaglandins, prostacyclins, leukotrienes and thromboxanes) trigger inflammation, redness, heat, swelling, and sometimes pain. These reactions are designed to reject the invaders and warn you that damage may have occurred to your body. But they can also lead to allergic or asthmatic reactions and other autoimmune responses.

The types of fat in your body can influence which of these eicosanoids are sent into battle. Omega-3 fats (fish oil, flax, etc.) will favor the less intense prostaglandins, whereas *omega-6 fats* (most cooking/frying oils) tend to *amplify inflammation*.

ALLERGIES

Allergies represent a condition in which your immune system identifies a substance (internal or external) as alien to your body and attempts to disable and/or quarantine it before it can harm your system.

The mobilization of that allergic/immune response creates inflammation. And inflammation causes a host of other problems.

When the substance is harmful to you (toxins, bacteria or viruses, for example), that inflammatory response helps you fight off the attacker and heal from an attack.

But when the substances are ordinary, non-threatening pollens or foods, this immune response is unwanted and harmful.

You can be allergic or sensitive to any number of things, including:

- Pollens and spores
- Foods
- Plants (poison ivy, etc.)
- Perfumes, dyes, etc.
- Hormones

HORMONE ALLERGIES

Yes, you can be allergic to your own hormones! Studies have found the presence of antibodies to natural human estrogen and progesterone in women with a variety of symptoms that fluctuate with their menstrual cycles

Although the idea has been around since studies first confirmed the phenomenon in the 1920s, still only a handful of practitioners are testing and treating patients for hormone allergies today. To be honest, we need a lot more research to understand the mechanisms at work and to refine the testing and treatment methods.

The most common suspected hormone allergy is to progesterone. This is ironic, since progesterone is the hormone that dampens the immune response during pregnancy to keep your body from attacking your baby as if it were a foreign object.

Some women may be allergic to estrogen as well, and perhaps other hormones that have not yet been studied.

How do hormone allergies present themselves? According to doctors who are working in this largely uncharted territory, the following reactions are just a sampling, though, as with other allergies, the symptoms can vary dramatically from person to person:

- PMS/PMDD
- Exaggerated traditional nasal allergies
- Asthma flare-ups
- Headaches/migraines
- Infertility
- Pain/fibromyalgia
- Inflammatory disease flares

Dr. Jonathan Wright—who is considered the father of bio-identical HRT—observed in his practice that about half of patients with PMS were not ovulating regularly and could be helped by supplementing progesterone during cycles when they did not ovulate (i.e., were not producing progesterone).

The other half of Dr. Wright's PMS patients appeared to actually be *allergic to their own progesterone* and would see their symptoms increase shortly before their periods.

Dr. Wright uses desensitization therapy in a manner similar to that of an allergist, exposing your body to the offending substance until you develop a tolerance to it.

But testing for hormone allergies can be tricky.

For those having a severe asthma attack, a few drops of highly diluted progesterone placed under the tongue may stop the attack in its tracks within seconds, suggesting an obvious hormone allergy connection.

For others, the symptoms may be more subtle or subjective: a pain becomes somewhat less bothersome or itching eases up upon receiving the diluted progesterone drops or injection.

For most, the diagnosis may take much more deliberation in order to rule out more obvious causes and to track symptoms against measured hormone levels.

Toxins

Toxins can include **heavy metals, food additives and drugs, as well as disease-causing bacteria, viruses, parasites and fungi**.

Among the most disturbing toxins in our world today are the **neurotoxins** we are exposed to from industrial and household chemicals, pesticides, therapeutic and recreational drugs, refined/processed foods, and cosmetic ingredients. These toxins can damage the brain and nervous system.

Among the worst of the neurotoxins are additives used in many "junk" foods—like those cheesy orange snacks that don't resemble anything in nature. They are considered **excitotoxins**, which can *overstimulate brain cells until they die!*

Monosodium glutamate (MSG), and the artificial sweetener, aspartame (NutraSweet/Equal), are perhaps the most well-known excitotoxins.

Aspartame breaks down into formaldehyde and formic acid (the toxin that gives fire ants their sting) in your system, neither of which was ever meant to be in your body.

And there are lots more excitotoxins, including a couple of them that sound harmless but are far from it. *(We'll give you a list of excitotoxin names at the end of this section.)*

Product labels can technically claim these are "natural." For example, glutamate is natural: it is the most abundant neurotransmitter in the brain. But your brain was never meant to be exposed to the extreme levels of glutamate produced by these food additives.

These toxins can cause migraines, seizures, sleep disruption, obesity, endocrine disorders and neurodegenerative diseases such as ALS, Alzheimer's, Parkinson's and Huntington's diseases. In children, they can forever alter their brains and predispose them to a range of conditions, especially obesity.

So do your homework, read product labels, and try to keep toxins out of your body. Your purification/detoxification system may be no match for the onslaught of these tasty manmade poisons.

TYPES OF TOXINS

There are many substances you may be exposed to that act as toxins in your body. They can include:

- **Food additives**. Flavor enhancers in foods can overstimulate the brain and cause brain cells to die.
- **Pesticides**. These may be absorbed through the skin, inhaled, or consumed in foods/drinks.
- **Xenohormones**. These are chemical substances in plastics, drugs and other sources that act on your body's cells as if they were hormones but are much harder to break down and excrete. They may include synthetic hormones injected into meat animals to fatten them up.
- **Heavy metals**. Your body can accumulate these through exposure to old lead-based paint, lead pipes, pesticides, mercury exposure from old thermometers, aluminum from cookware, table salt and antiperspirants, etc.
- **Parasites.** Tape worms, round worms and pinworms are only a few of the parasites that can take up residence in your body.

FOOD ADDITIVE TOXINS (EXCITOTOXINS)

The toxins in processed foods—substances that can literally
excite brain cells to death—may be called by many names,
including those shown below:

- MSG (monosodium glutamate)
- Aspartame (NutraSweet, Equal, etc.)
- Caseinate
- Autolyzed or hydrolyzed protein
- Autolyzed yeast extract
- Soy isolates, soy protein concentrate
- Beef/chicken broth (which contains MSG)
- Natural flavor/flavoring
- Vegetable protein extract

Symptoms of Toxicity

Toxicity symptoms can vary dramatically, depending upon the
toxin and the degree of exposure. But some of the most common
symptoms of toxicity are:

- Headache
- Nausea, vomiting
- Constipation or diarrhea
- Weight loss
- Dizziness
- Anemia
- Joint pain
- Weakness, loss of coordination
- Cough

TESTING FOR TOXINS

Hair analysis may help reveal the presence of heavy metal toxins in your system. Blood and stool testing can identify other toxins.

Detoxification

Your body has its own detoxification processes to trap toxins and (ideally) flush them out of your system. But when your body needs help detoxifying, a number of methods can facilitate the process.

NATURAL DETOXIFICATION

Detoxification occurs naturally in your body through a few key systems and organs:

- Lymphatic system
- Liver
- Kidneys
- Sweat glands

In many cases, you may be able to help those systems and organs do their jobs.

THE LYMPHATIC SYSTEM

The lymphatic system runs through virtually every part of your body. It is a network of vessels and nodes that contains nearly three times more fluid (lymph) than the bloodstream.

But you rarely think about your lymphatic system...until you have an infection. That's when you can feel the swollen lymph nodes in your neck or armpits or groin. That swelling indicates the lymphatic system has detected an invader (a virus, bacteria, parasites, toxic chemicals or metals, or even cancer) and is working hard to stop it from invading the rest of your body.

What most of us don't know is that—unlike the vascular system, which uses the heart to pump blood around—the lymphatic system has no pump. The only way to move lymph—and the junk it traps—is to move your body.

That's why even moderate exercise can be so beneficial to your immune system. Just doing housework, bending and lifting and stretching in different directions, helps move lymphatic fluid and toxins through the pipeline toward the kidneys, liver or sweat glands for removal.

See Detoxification Solutions in Chapter 21.

LIVER

The liver is the workhorse of the purification system, which is why it often takes the brunt of our typical lifestyle abuses...like eating junk food, drinking alcohol or using pesticides.

The liver's primary job is to produce powerful enzymes that can convert fat-soluble toxins into water-soluble form that can be excreted in the urine or feces.

Fat-soluble toxins are the most dangerous because they can hide in fat for years, leaching out their poisons into your bloodstream over time. That's why you may have to work even harder to get them out of your system.

KIDNEYS

The kidneys help your body remove water-soluble wastes.

They also regulate the body's acid/base (pH) balance and electrolytes, and remove fluid from tissues.

And as we learned earlier, they help regulate blood pressure.

Because sediments (of calcium and other materials) can accumulate in the kidneys and form stones that cause severe pain, you should drink plenty of plain water to flush out sediments.

SWEAT GLANDS

Sweating helps your body rid itself of toxins such as alcohol, nicotine (from cigarettes), and sodium. Sweating is especially effective in removing toxins that have been stored in fat cells, which may be impossible to excrete any other way.

EXTERNAL DETOXIFICATION

You may occasionally need a little help getting rid of extra doses of toxins you've consumed or absorbed through your skin or breathed in.

Several methods can help force these substances out of your body, including:

- Chelation (for heavy metals)
- Cleansing
- Lymphatic stimulation
- Sauna

We'll describe detoxification methods in more detail, along with all the recommended solutions, in Part D, next.

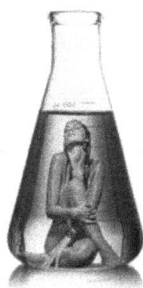

PART D: **SOLUTIONS**

SOLUTIONS NOTES

Use this page to make notes about the solutions you think may
be especially helpful to you.

18| Solutions (General)

This chapter will explore all the recommended non-hormonal, non-vitamin solutions (minerals, herbals, lifestyle choices, etc.), and will provide guidance as to how to benefit from them.

Remember: The content here is for informational purposes only. You should work with a trusted healthcare professional when implementing any wellness solutions.

The following three chapters (19-21) of Part D will cover vitamin solutions, hormonal solutions, and solution protocols (combinations of solutions that work synergistically to prevent or reverse a common problem).

The minerals, herbs and other solutions are listed here in alphabetical order.

Azo/Phenazopyridine

- *See Urinary Tract Solutions in Chapter 21.*

Black Cohosh

Of all the herbal solutions recommended for reducing hot flashes and preserving bone, the most effective non-estrogenic option may be black cohosh.

Unlike soy and red clover products that contain plant estrogens (phytoestrogens), black cohosh has no estrogenic effect. In fact, it's not clear exactly why it helps reduce hot flashes, but it does. Black cohosh is one of the few herbal treatments that have been recommended by American gynecologists, though its effects are much milder than those of estrogen.

- *See Estrogen in Chapter 20: Hormonal Solutions.*

Black cohosh may also help reduce ringing in the ears (tinnitus), especially when used with zinc.

Broccoli, Cauliflower, Cabbage, etc.

Cruciferous vegetables (broccoli, cauliflower, cabbage, Brussels sprouts, etc.) are among the most important secret weapons in every royal diet.

BENEFITS

- **Broad spectrum cancer prevention/fighting**. Cruciferous veggies help prevent *nearly every kind of cancer including deadly pancreatic cancer!*

- **Prevent estrogen-related cancers, alter the 2/16 ratio.** The substances in these veggies influence how your body breaks down natural estrogens in your body and encourages the formation of the beneficial 2-version instead of the more cancer-prone 16-version. *(See The 2/16 Ratio in Chapter 14.)*

- **Prevent/reverse heart disease in diabetics.** Studies have shown that broccoli may help reverse the kind of heart damage that is caused by diabetes.

- **May reduce anxiety**. Although there is currently no explanation for it, some women find that broccoli, eaten at least every 3 or 4 days can help prevent anxiety attacks or reduce the severity of anxiety.

HOW TO USE THEM

- **Consume at least 5 regular (or 2-3 large) servings a week.** You don't need to eat them every day. Just try to include an extra-large serving of cruciferous veggies in your diet about every 3 days to create a sustained level of protection in your system.

- **Vary the preparation method.** Because some of their nutrients are released when the fibers are broken (in chewing or chopping) and others are released in cooking, it's best to include both raw and cooked (steamed) variations of these veggies in your diet each week. Just be sure to undercook them to preserve their nutrients.

- **Frozen vs. fresh.** Some so-called "fresh" produce may sit in warehouses or trucks or store shelves for long periods of time, losing their nutrients before ever reaching your home. On the other hand, frozen veggies like broccoli and cauliflower may be preserved at their nutritional peak and may deliver more nutrients than comparable fresh products.

- **Sprouts vs. mature.** Broccoli sprouts that are 3-4 days old have at least 20 times the nutrients of mature broccoli. So if you grow them yourself or buy organic sprouts from local suppliers, you can enjoy the same benefits by sprinkling some on a salad or sandwich a few times a week.

WHAT YOU NEED TO KNOW

- **Supplements are available.** If you absolutely can't stand to eat any of the cruciferous veggies, you can find supplements that deliver the key substances in broccoli and its kin — primarily indole-3-carbinol (I3C), sulforaphane and DIM. Just remember that the natural foods (if they are fresh and grown in fertile soil) may deliver the bigger benefits.

Calcium

You probably know that you need calcium (among other things) to make strong bones. But you may not need to go out of your way to supplement calcium if you have a healthy diet.

BENEFITS

- Helps build bones.
- Supports nerve and muscle function.
- Enables formation of long-term memories.
- (With magnesium and potassium) helps control blood pressure.

HOW TO GET IT

Foods that contain lots of calcium include:
- Milk, yogurt, cheese
- Broccoli (and other cruciferous veggies), spinach, collard greens
- Oranges
- Salmon
- Peas, peanuts, black beans

You can also get calcium cheaply in the form of calcium-based antacids, but that's not the best approach.

WHAT YOU NEED TO KNOW

- **Too much calcium can be harmful**. If you over-supplement or inadvertently get too much calcium (in calcium-fortified foods and drinks), you may end up with white splotches in your fingernails, constipation, dry mouth, headache or even depression. More important, the excess calcium can end up in your joints, causing pain and possibly leading to arthritis.

- **Take it with other nutrients**. You need to balance calcium with proper levels of potassium, magnesium and vitamin D3 for optimal effectiveness.

- **Calcium can alter body pH and impact digestion**. When you take calcium, you reduce the acidity of your system. For those who have what appears to be heartburn/reflux caused by too little stomach acid, taking calcium supplements will make this situation worse unless you also supplement HCL and pepsin.

- **There are two common forms of calcium**: calcium citrate and calcium carbonate. If you have low stomach acid (HCL) it's better to take calcium *citrate*. Calcium *carbonate* contains a higher proportion of calcium, but it is absorbed best when taken with food (assuming you have enough HCL).

Calorie Restriction

- *See Longevity Solutions in Chapter 21.*

Carnosine

Carnosine is one of those supplements that help you reverse the damage done to your body by toxins—especially excitotoxins.

Your body normally makes carnosine from a couple of amino acids, but you produce less of it as you age. Carnosine can help slow aging, and may be even more important for protection against neurotoxin brain damage.

BENEFITS

- Chelates (attaches to and removes) heavy metals.
- Promotes healthy blood sugar.
- Slows aging, especially in the skin (improves elasticity, reduces wrinkles).
- Is a powerful antioxidant.

- Improves endurance.
- May help prevent cataracts, Alzheimer's disease.

HOW TO USE IT

- Carnosine (or L-carnosine) is available in most health food stores.
- To reverse aging, you may need to take 500 to 750 mg twice a day (1000-1500 mg/day).

Chromium

Chromium can be effective in reducing sugar and carb cravings and aiding in overall weight loss and fat burning.

HOW TO USE IT

- Chromium picolinate is available at most health food stores, sometimes combined with other substances. It's best to avoid combo products where possible, or at least be aware of the effects the other ingredients may have.
- Take 5000-6000 mcg (5-6 mg) per day till cravings stop, then reduce dose to 1000 mcg (1 mg) per day.

WHAT YOU NEED TO KNOW

- Chromium may be toxic in high doses of 70,000 mcg (70 mg) and above. However, to get this much, you would have to take a whole bottle or more of capsules in one sitting.
- Chromium picolinate supplements typically come in 250-500 mcg capsules. So to achieve a 5000 mcg dose, you would have to take 10 of the 500 mcg capsules a day or 20 of the 250 mcg capsules per day until cravings subside, then settle into a dose of 2 of the 500 mcg (or 4 of the 250 mcg) capsules per day.

- The jury is still out regarding the effectiveness of chromium for dramatic weight loss. However, most studies have used far lower doses than those suggested here.

Cimetidine

Although few people realize it, the heartburn drug cimetidine (Tagamet) doesn't work very well for acid reflux, but it may be a life saver for those who have been diagnosed with colon or stomach cancer or may be at risk for these diseases.

Many studies, starting in the 1970s and continuing today, have demonstrated this drug's ability to prevent tumor metastasis and dramatically improve the survival rate for patients with these cancers. A 2006 report in the *International Journal of Oncology* describes some of the latest confirmations of cimetidine's benefits.

BENEFITS

- May be more effective than chemotherapy alone for colon, stomach and lung cancer, as well as squamous cell carcinoma and melanoma.

HOW TO USE IT

- Doses of 800-1000 mg/day are relatively harmless and have been used successfully to prevent tumor metastases. This dosage may also prevent cancer in those who are at higher risk, whether genetically or due to other factors.

WHAT YOU NEED TO KNOW

- Generic cimetadine is available over the counter. Shop around and look online for the most affordable brands.

CoQ10/Ubiquinol

When the roads you travel on get potholes, repair crews come along to fill them with concrete or asphalt. Your body is just like that. CoQ10 works with cholesterol to repair normal damage to various organs, especially the heart and liver. If your CoQ10 (and/or cholesterol) is low, your body may not have the filler materials with which to repair your cells.

BENEFITS

CoQ10 supplementation has proven beneficial in a number of ways:

- Helps prevent breast and prostate cancer; reduces the recurrence of breast cancer.
- Reduces liver damage in those taking statins for cholesterol.
- Is a powerful antioxidant (50 times more potent than vitamin E).
- Repairs cells and keeps cell membranes elastic (prevents or reduces inflammation).
- Prevents heart disease.
- Is a vital nutrient for cells, with highest levels in the heart, liver and kidneys.
- Helps maintain healthy blood sugar levels.
- Helps prevent migraine headaches.
- Preserves vision.
- Supports immune function.
- Slows progression of Parkinson's disease.
- Has significant anti-aging effects on virtually all cells, especially skin.
- May reduce blood sugar levels in some individuals.

COQ10 AND CHOLESTEROL-LOWERING DRUGS (STATINS)

It's best to avoid taking statins unless absolutely necessary. (Remember, your body needs cholesterol.) But if you do take statins, you should know that they deplete CoQ10, break down cell walls, and can cause liver damage, numbness and/or pain, muscle wasting, and kidney blockage as a result.

So if you take statins, at least be sure to supplement your diet with CoQ10.

HOW TO USE COQ10

Ubiquinol is a form of CoQ10 that is roughly 1.5 times more potent (more bioavailable) than regular CoQ10 (ubiquinone).

So a 100 mg capsule of ubiquinol is equivalent to 150 mg of regular CoQ10/ubiquinone.

TYPICAL DOSE

- *For overall health* (those who are not taking statins): 100-150 mg of ubiquinol per day (or 150-225 mg regular CoQ10/ubiquinone).
- *For those taking statins or those who seek the anti-aging effects of CoQ10*: 200-300 mg ubiquinol per day (or 300-450 mg regular CoQ10/ubiquinone).

Curcumin

Curcumin is the substance that gives spices like turmeric and curry their bright orange color. Curcumin is one of the most potent natural antioxidants, anti-inflammatories and cancer fighters.

BENEFITS

- Prevents/fights many diseases (including Alzheimer's, cancer, atherosclerosis).

- Reduces inflammation.

- Prevents/reduces allergies.

- Thins blood, prevents plaque in cardiovascular system.

HOW TO USE IT

- You can use turmeric or curry in foods.

- For medicinal purposes, take 60-100 mg curcumin 1-2 times per day.

D-Mannose

D-mannose is a type of sugar that can help you get rid of certain urinary tract infections (UTIs) quickly and easily.

- *See Urinary Tract Solutions in Chapter 21.*

Electrolytes

Electrolytes are substances your body needs in order to maintain proper electrical conductivity. When you are low in electrolytes, you may find that your muscles begin to misfire and twitch or cramp. Exercise or illness (and vomiting) with insufficient hydration can deplete electrolytes.

Electrolytes include:
- Potassium
- Sodium
- Calcium and magnesium

Many sports drinks help replace these electrolytes.

WHAT YOU NEED TO KNOW

If you have sodium-sensitive high blood pressure, you may want to avoid sports drinks that are high in sodium.

Ellagic Acid

- *See Quercetin and Ellagic Acid.*

Feverfew

The herb feverfew, especially with 5-HTP (a precursor to serotonin), has been shown in several small studies and a meta analysis to be effective in reducing the number and severity of migraine headaches.

BENEFITS

- May prevent or reduce severity of migraine headaches.
- May also be effective (especially in combination with other herbs) in reducing the inflammation of rheumatoid arthritis.

HOW TO USE IT

- Look for feverfew supplements that are standardized to contain at least 0.2% parthenolide (the active ingredient).
- For migraines, take 100 - 300 mg, up to 4 times daily (standardized to contain 0.2 - 0.4% parthenolides).

WHAT YOU NEED TO KNOW

- Feverfew may act as a blood thinner, so use with caution or avoid if you are already on blood thinners.
- The most dramatic results for migraine prevention come from studies using feverfew twice a day continuously.
- Using feverfew with magnesium and vitamin B2 may cut the frequency of migraines by half.

Ginger

For those prone to motion sickness and other causes of nausea, this little herbal remedy can be life saver. The crew of TV's *MythBusters* showed this natural substance to be at least as effective as diphenhydramine (Dramamine) in curbing nausea, with fewer side effects.

I personally swear by ginger to prevent motion sickness and reduce nausea caused by anesthesia and illness (at least in situations where I can keep something in my stomach long enough for it to take effect).

HOW TO USE IT

- **For motion sickness.** Take 2 capsules of ginger (500 mg each) with water about 30 minutes prior to departure on a plane or other mode of travel. Be prepared to add doses (1-2 capsules) at 3- to 4-hour intervals to sustain the anti-nausea effects through longer journeys.

- **For general nausea.** You need to catch it early enough that you can keep the ginger in your stomach for at least 30 minutes. If you cannot keep anything down, you may need a prescription anti-nausea suppository (Phenergan/promethazine, etc.) initially to stop the vomiting cycle.

WHAT YOU NEED TO KNOW

- Ginger's anti-nausea effects may only last 3-4 hours, so be prepared to take additional "booster" doses every few hours, whether two capsules or just one, throughout the duration of your journey.

- It's best to take ginger with a little bit of food and plenty of water/liquid, otherwise you may experience some heartburn.

Ginkgo Biloba

Ginkgo biloba is traditionally known for enhancing memory and improving circulation.

Ginkgo can also help reduce ringing in the ears (tinnitus), especially when taken with zinc. And it can help prevent or treat vertigo and Meniere's disease.

- Take 40 mg, 3 times per day of standardized 50:1 extract.

Glucosamine, Chondroitin, MSM

It is rare to hear a surgeon endorse the use of over-the-counter remedies, but for the relief of joint inflammation and pain, the combination of glucosamine, chondroitin and MSM has proven to be an effective complementary treatment accepted by many mainstream doctors.

HOW TO USE IT

- Start out with 1500 mg of glucosamine and 1200 of chondroitin daily for 1- 2 months. If this initial dosage proves effective, you can cut back to a maintenance dosage of 1000 mg of glucosamine and 800 of chondroitin or less.

WHAT YOU NEED TO KNOW

- Avoid taking glucosamine if you are allergic to shellfish.

- If you are diabetic, watch for elevation of blood sugar.

- Avoid these products if you are taking blood thinners (such as Coumadin), as they may increase the risk of bleeding.

- MSM is also beneficial in reducing the symptoms of irritable bowel syndrome (IBS) and leaky gut.

Glutamine (L-Glutamine)

L-glutamine (or just *glutamine*) is one of the 20 amino acid your body makes. It is the second most important source of cellular energy after glucose (blood sugar).

Not to be confused with:

- *Glutamate*—the neurotransmitter whose effects are dangerously elevated by excitotoxins like MSG (monosodium glutamate) in prepared foods.
- *Glutathione*—the antioxidant made inside your body that you may supplement for detoxification purposes.

Glutamine is the most abundant free amino acid in your body, but your internal supplies can burn up rapidly when your system is coping with trauma (injury/burn, illness, surgery, etc.).

GLUTAMINE BENEFITS

Glutamine can be helpful in a number of ways:

- Helps speed up the body's healing processes (especially the gut) following trauma. (Some hospitals routinely supplement glutamine for surgery patients.)
- Strengthens immune system.
- Supports a healthy gut and maintains gut barrier to block out toxins.
- Protects liver.
- Helps maintain stable blood sugar levels.
- Promotes development of muscle, increases endurance.
- Helps prevent or reduce the peripheral neuropathy (numbness of hands/feet) that occurs in diabetics and those taking platinum-based chemotherapy.
- May help fight rheumatoid arthritis and other autoimmune diseases.

HOW TO USE IT

- Glutamine is typically available in powder form from most health food stores.

- Take 10 grams per day mixed in a drink or in food until wounds are healed or illness is cured.

- For chemo, begin taking glutamine the day before chemo and continue taking for 3-4 weeks after the last platinum-based chemo treatment.

WHAT YOU NEED TO KNOW

- Once nerve damage is done, you may not be able to reverse it, so prevention is critical.

- Bodybuilders have been using glutamine for decades to accelerate muscle repair after an intense workout.

- Glutamine does not dissolve fully in liquids, so if you don't like the gritty texture in drinks, you may want to mix it with grainy foods like cereal, oatmeal or applesauce.

- Cooking destroys glutamine, so add it to cooked foods only after they have cooled a bit.

- Do not use glutamine without a doctor's guidance if you have liver or kidney disease or are sensitive to MSG.

Glutathione

Glutathione is an endogenous (made inside the body) antioxidant that can also play a key role in detoxification.

BENEFITS

It serves a number of purposes:
- Neutralizes free radicals that can lead to cancer.
- Detoxifies foreign substances (especially heavy metals).
- Supports the immune, nervous, and gastrointestinal systems and lung function.

- Supports various metabolic processes.

HOW TO USE IT

For extreme detoxification purposes, your doctor may administer glutathione intravenously. You may also be able to stimulate the natural production of glutathione by using acupuncture or nanotechnology patches that function in a similar manner to that of acupuncture.

Two supplements that can help increase glutathione levels are:

- SAMe and Milk thistle/silymarin

WHAT YOU NEED TO KNOW

- Although glutathione can protect against cancer, if you already have cancer, high doses of glutathione may reduce the effectiveness of chemotherapy drugs.

Hawthorn Berry

Hawthorn berry may be effective in helping to reduce heart disease risks.

BENEFITS

- Reduces blood pressure
- Lowers cholesterol

HOW TO USE IT

Some cases of high blood pressure respond to hawthorn berry— with or without potassium supplementation.

- A dose of 900 to 1200 mg a day may be sufficient to reduce blood pressure to normal levels.

Hydrochloric Acid (HCL) and Pepsin

If you have too little HCL in your stomach and suffer what appear to be symptoms of heartburn or reflux, the easiest solution is to take an HCL pill at the beginning of each meal.

HOW TO USE IT

- Betaine HCL is a product that contains between 300 and 650 mg of HCL, sometimes paired with pepsin, a critical enzyme that works with HCL to break down your food.

- Some people may only need a little, others may need a lot.

- Take it at the beginning of each meal or snack.

- *See Chapter 15: Nutritional/Digestive Processes; and Chapter 22: Resources.*

Iodine

Iodine—prepared as a saturated solution of potassium iodide (SSKI), Lugol's solution, or other combinations of iodine and iodide—can be helpful for any number of purposes.

BENEFITS

- Reduces the density of fibrocystic breasts.
- May reduce the recurrence of breast cancer.
- May help prevent ovarian cysts.
- Supports thyroid function (in optimal doses).

HOW TO USE IT

- Take 5 mg of SSKI Tri-quench (6-8 drops in water) twice a day for 3 to 6 months to reduce density and pain of fibrocystic breasts or to treat ovarian cysts.

- If using Iodoral or Lugol's solution, follow the instructions of your healthcare advisor.

WHAT YOU NEED TO KNOW

- Be sure your healthcare team monitors your thyroid levels while you are taking any form of iodine, as too much can lower thyroid hormones.

Iron

For iron-deficiency anemia, the most effective solution is to take iron supplements.

Bad breath may be a symptom of iron deficiency anemia.

IDENTIFYING IRON-DEFICIENCY ANEMIA

If you've had a standard CBC blood test recently, you should be able to spot iron-deficiency anemia in the results listed beside "MCV."

MCV results that are *below* normal (indicating small red blood cells) suggest iron deficiency. (*Higher*-than-normal results suggest a vitamin B12 deficiency.)

WHAT YOU NEED TO KNOW

- Iron overload can lead to serious conditions such as diabetes or arthritis, so be sure to work with your healthcare advisor and monitor your bloodwork if you are taking iron.
- Postmenopausal women (who no longer experience monthly menstruation) may be more prone to iron overload.

Laxatives (Natural)

Cleansing procedures often include the use of a gentle laxative. You may also occasionally need to reverse a bout of constipation.

Two of the most common natural laxatives are:

- Prunes
- Senna (prepared as a tea or in herbal products)

L-glutamine

See Glutamine.

Lithium

Lithium is most famously known for its use as a prescription drug for treating bi-polar disorder. However, used in much smaller dosages, it can be helpful for supporting memory.

BENEFITS

- Protects neurons and the brain against damage from neurotoxins, stroke and age-related cognitive decline (and Alzheimer's). May also repair or rebuild brain cells.
- Reduces alcohol cravings.
- Reduces aggressiveness.

HOW TO USE IT

- Take 5 mg 3 times a day.

WHAT YOU NEED TO KNOW

- Lithium is an essential trace element your body needs. It is in the same family of minerals as sodium and potassium.
- A UC San Diego study of 27 Texas counties over 10 years showed that those counties whose drinking water contained 70-170 mcg of lithium per liter had significantly lower crime and suicide rates than counties with little or no lithium in the water. A 2009 Japanese study reported similar findings.

- Low-dose (5 to 20 mg) lithium is available over the counter from online pharmacies.

Lysine

Lysine is an amino acid that has been shown effective in shortening the duration of herpes simplex (cold sores/fever blisters) and herpes zoster (chickenpox, shingles) outbreaks.

HOW TO USE IT

- Take 1000 mg 3 times a day until the outbreak heals.
- You may experience extra benefits by adding the amino acid arginine.

Magnesium

Magnesium is a mineral that is essential for bone building and heart health.

BENEFITS

- Reduces risk of heart disease.
- Works with calcium to build bones.
- Protects against excitotoxins.
- Reduces inflammation.

HOW TO USE IT

- Take 400-800 mg per day (with calcium and vitamin D3 for optimal absorption and balance).

Malic Acid

Malic acid naturally occurs in various tart foods, especially apples.

BENEFITS

- Reduces the symptoms of fibromyalgia and chronic fatigue syndrome.

- Increases energy, decreases muscle fatigue.

- Boosts immune system.

- Serves as a chelation agent to help remove heavy metals, especially aluminum.

- May help prevent heartburn.

HOW TO USE IT

- Take 1200-1600 mg a day in supplements.

- As part of a cleanse, take 1-3 tablespoons of apple cider vinegar every few hours throughout the day.

Milk Thistle, Bupleurum

Milk thistle has long been known in folk medicine for its ability to protect and heal the liver. Bupleurum is an herb related to fennel and dill that works synergistically with milk thistle.

BENEFITS

- Help protect, cleanse and heal the liver.

- May reduce severity of cirrhosis, hepatitis.

- May help prevent liver cancer.

Omega Oils

You have surely heard that omega-3 oils are important to your health. But did you know that you also need omega-6 oils as well?

Both of these essential fatty acids (EFAs) support healthy brain and immune function and help regulate blood pressure.

Ideally, you would have an even balance of the two, or at most a 2:1 ratio of omega-6 to omega-3 oils (twice as much omega-6 as omega-3).

However, the typical Western diet may include as much as *15 times* more omega-6 than omega-3 oils. And that sets us up for any number of inflammatory diseases, especially heart disease.

The reason you hear such one-sided advice is that it is all too easy for us to get omega-6 oils (in fried/prepared foods, snacks and salad/cooking oils), but we have to work a lot harder to get an equal amount of omega-3 oils (in fish, flax).

OMEGA-3 OILS

Omega-3 oils reduce inflammation, and support heart health and immune function.

BENEFITS

Omega-3 oils help manage or reduce the severity of many conditions including: asthma, diabetes, arthritis, osteoporosis, some cancers, skin disorders, high cholesterol, high blood pressure, attention disorders, depression, macular degeneration.

HOW TO GET THEM

- You can find omega-3 oils in whole grains, green leafy vegetables, nuts and seeds (Brazil nuts, mustard & pumpkin seeds, walnuts, flaxseed, etc.), and oils (rapeseed, hempseed, chia seed, canola, flaxseed).

- Although fish provides the most abundant source of omega-3 oils, many fish contain high levels of mercury, which is a heavy metal and a neurotoxin. If you eat fish, be sure to do your research to learn which ones have the least amount of mercury.

- If you choose fish oil supplements, make sure they are high quality and do not contain mercury.
- For general health, supplement 1000 mg or more omega-3 oils per day.

WHAT YOU NEED TO KNOW

- Fish oils can be stinky, both in their capsules and when they come back to haunt you as gas. Krill oil delivers all the benefits of fish oil without the gas.
- To relieve the symptoms of arthritis, you may need huge doses (6-12 pills a day). Ask your doctor about prescription omega-3 fish oil, which is highly concentrated.

OMEGA-6 OILS

Omega-6s have gotten a bad reputation because they promote inflammation. But if you'll recall the chapter on purification systems (immunity and detoxification), inflammation is an important function of the immune system that helps our bodies guard against and remove toxins and other invaders.

The trouble comes when we consume dozens of times more of these pro-inflammatory fats than of the anti-inflammatory omega-3s. Fried foods are notoriously high in omega-6 oils.

HOW TO GET THEM

There are good and bad omega-6 oils. Here are some of the best:
- Olive oil
- Wheat germ
- Raw nuts and seeds (pistachios, grape, pumpkin, etc.)
- Sesame, safflower, sunflower, cottonseed oils

WHAT YOU NEED TO KNOW

- When you cook or fry with any kind of oil (omega-3 or 6), be aware that high heat can oxidize them. These oxidized oils can damage your cardiovascular system and may cause the kind of cellular damage that can lead to cancer.

- Although coconut oil is not technically an omega-3 oil, it provides healthy fats in the same family. More importantly, it can be stored longer without turning rancid and can tolerate higher temperatures without oxidizing, so you may want to choose this oil for pan browning and frying. Be sure to get cold-pressed coconut oils and avoid those that may be hydrogenated into trans-fats.

OMEGA-9 OILS

Omega-9 oils also play a role in preventing heart disease and promoting healthy immune function. But you don't need to do anything special to get them: your body will make omega-9 fats if you are consuming plenty of omega-3 and omega-6 oils.

Phosphatidyl Serine

Phosphatidyl serine is a substance normally found in the body that helps support healthy brain function. It can also help reduce stress-related cortisol damage.

BENEFITS

- Supports memory and cognition, increases the neurotransmitters acetylcholine and dopamine in the brain.

- Reduces cortisol stress damage.

- May reduce depression.

HOW TO GET IT

- Take 200 to 300 mg per day.

Potassium

Potassium is the third most abundant mineral in your body. It is important for building bone, regulating nerve transmission and maintaining blood pressure.

BENEFITS

- Enables healthy muscle contractions, promotes muscle strength (including heart muscle).
- Prevents muscle cramps (though too *high* and too *low* potassium can cause cramps).
- Helps regulate blood pressure in balance with sodium.
- Prevents stroke.
- Helps stabilize blood sugar (with sodium).
- Reduces the effects of stress.
- Helps maintain proper fluid balance. Is an important electrolyte.
- Supports healthy metabolism.

WHAT YOU NEED TO KNOW

- Both high and low potassium levels can cause muscle cramps. Be sure you know which is the cause before taking potassium to stop cramps.
- If your foot or leg cramps are the result of potassium deficiency, you may reverse them within 15-30 minutes by taking as little as 30-50 mg.
- Potassium supplements are typically packaged in 99 mg pills. (I don't know why it's 99 and not 100.)

- Although most of us have been led to believe that sodium (salt) is always bad for those with high blood pressure, what is more important is the balance between sodium and potassium. Some patients with high blood pressure may simply have to add potassium to their diets and not have to cut back on salt. Be sure to check with your doctor for guidance, because not all cases of hypertension respond to potassium.

Probiotics

Probiotics are supplements that replace the friendly microorganisms in your digestive tract that may have been killed or compromised by stress, illness or antibiotic use.

BENEFITS

- Prevent or reverse leaky gut syndrome, protecting you from toxins that may otherwise leak through intestinal walls into your bloodstream before they can be disabled and eliminated properly by the digestive system.
- May prevent irritable bowel syndrome and colitis.
- Improve immune system, help fight infection.
- Help prevent diarrhea and urinary infections.
- May help prevent colon cancer.
- Help lower blood pressure and cholesterol.
- Improve mineral absorption.

HOW TO GET THEM

Many probiotics (such as bifidobacterium and acidophilus) are included as live cultures in yogurt and certain supplements.

The most common probiotic is lactic acid bacteria (lactobacillus), which helps those who are lactose intolerant to enjoy dairy products.

WHAT YOU NEED TO KNOW

Because probiotics are living creatures, certain methods of processing or transporting them may inadvertently kill the cultures.

Lactobacillus products, for example, may need to be refrigerated throughout the life of the product in order to keep the cultures alive. The most reliable way to ensure you are getting live lactobacillus cultures may be to purchase products (such as Lactinex) through your local pharmacy. Although no prescription is required, the pharmacy ensures these products have been handled properly and kept cool.

HOW TO USE THEM

- If you have been on antibiotics, you should finish out the course before starting on probiotics to restore your GI tract.

- However, if your antibiotics are causing diarrhea and stomach upset, you may want to include probiotics each day to calm your gut, even though the drugs will kill them off.

- Once you are finished with your antibiotics, or if you are simply trying to reverse damage done to your gut over time, you may begin supplementing probiotics daily. You may need two weeks or a month of daily supplements.

- To promote healthy diversity, you may supplement more than one kind of probiotic bacteria.

Quercetin and Ellagic Acid

Quercetin and ellagic acid are flavanoids that have significant anti-cancer properties. They are found primarily in fruits (grapes, pomegranates, red raspberries, cranberries, blueberries, strawberries) as well as walnuts, green and black tea, broccoli and tomatoes.

BENEFITS

Together, these two substances have proven effective in suppressing or reducing cancers, especially leukemia.

ELLAGIC ACID

- Shown to reduce atherosclerosis (hardening of the arteries) by 1000%.
- Restores normal cell death (apoptosis) of cancer cells.
- Prevents carcinogens from binding to and damaging DNA.

QUERCETIN

- Is considered a plant estrogen; has some of the same effects as estrogen (i.e., it may help reduce hot flashes, slow bone loss, etc.).
- Prevents the antioxidant vitamin C from oxidizing.
- Helps prevent cataracts.
- Promotes skin elasticity.
- Kills viruses, especially with vitamin C.
- Reduces allergies (acts as an antihistamine).
- Stimulates bile for proper digestion.
- Helps prevent nerve, eye and kidney damage in diabetics.

HOW TO GET THEM

- Both can be obtained from citrus fruits and berries.
- Quercetin can also be found in onions, apples, red wine, and green tea.
- Supplements are not very effective sources of ellagic acid. The best sources are fresh or frozen berries/fruits and walnuts. Mix them into smoothies each day for maximum benefits.

- Quercetin is typically supplemented at around 100-250 mg/day.
- Quercetin is sometimes combined with bromelain, which also aids digestion (by breaking down proteins) and reduces inflammation and bruising.

Relora

Relora is an herbal product that reduces cortisol and helps prevent the damage that stress causes. It is the main ingredient in certain weight loss products that aim to reduce belly fat and insulin resistance.

BENEFITS

- Reduces anxiety, promotes relaxation.
- Reduces cortisol.
- May support sleep.
- May help reduce belly fat, increase insulin sensitivity.

Resveratrol

Resveratrol is the substance in red wine that we've been hearing so much about lately. It has a number of terrific benefits.

BENEFITS

Resveratrol is proving to be a near-miraculous substance that...
- Prevents cancer (especially breast and ovarian).
- Prevents heart disease, balances cholesterol.
- Speeds up metabolism.
- Is a powerful antioxidant.
- Increases overall life span in a manner similar to that of calorie restriction. *(See Longevity Solutions in Chapter 21.)*
- Softens skin, reduces wrinkles.
- Reduces bloating.

- Increases athletic endurance.
- Normalizes cholesterol levels and blood pressure.
- May help reduce irritable bowel syndrome (IBS).
- May improve vision.

HOW TO USE IT

- To get health and skin benefits, some experts say you need about 20-50 mg of pure resveratrol per day.
- Many products may show higher dosages on the front of the package. Look on the ingredients list to find the actual amount of resveratrol you will get from each capsule.
- Some recommend working up from dosages of about 25 mg a day to 500 mg a day over a period of 6 weeks (25, 100, 250, 500), increasing the dose every two weeks to minimize the side effects.

WHAT YOU NEED TO KNOW

- Resveratrol thins the blood as effectively as aspirin. Do not use it if you are taking blood thinners of any kind, including aspirin, without consulting with your doctor.
- Initial side effects can include: a buzzed, hyper feeling or anxiety; insomnia; increased blood pressure; diarrhea and/or stomach cramps. And it may temporarily increase inflammation. These should be minimal with lower doses and should fade as your body adjusts to the increasing doses.
- Normal resveratrol is processed out of your body in about 9-10 hours. So it may be best to use 2 or 3 small doses (15 mg each, for example) divided up throughout the day to sustain the benefits.
- Some recommend using trans-resveratrol, because it is the most bioavailable form of the nutrient.

- Muscadine grapes are the most beneficial of all grapes, containing more resveratrol and antioxidants than red grapes. And they are the only grapes containing ellagic acid. *(See Quercetin and Ellagic Acid.)*

SAMe

SAMe is a substance produced in the liver that is essential for cellular growth and repair and for the production of neurotransmitters.

BENEFITS

SAMe has a few key benefits:

- Increases glutathione, which promotes detoxification.
- Elevates mood, reduces mild depression.
- Shown to reduce the severity of post-partum depression as effectively as prescription antidepressants, but works faster and has none of the negative side effects.
- May help prevent Alzheimer's disease.
- Helps protect the liver and fight liver disease.

Selenium

Selenium is an antioxidant that we should be getting from our food. However, the soil in which much of our food is grown may be depleted of its nutrients, including selenium, and we can become deficient in selenium.

Many of the benefits of selenium supplementation are actually the result of reversing our selenium deficiencies.

BENEFITS

- Improves vision.

- Helps remove (chelates) heavy metal toxins, including mercury.

- (With vitamin E) helps prevent pancreatic cancer.

- (With vitamins C, E and beta carotene) helps prevent numerous other cancers (including breast, esophageal, stomach, prostate, liver and bladder).

- (With vitamins A and E) can reduce the toxicity of chemotherapy.

HOW TO USE IT

- The typical dose is 200 mcg a day.

St. John's Wort

Although it has not been found to be effective in treating major depression, St. John's Wort does provide some mood-elevating benefits for those with milder forms of depression.

WHAT YOU NEED TO KNOW

- St. John's wort can interact with certain drugs (including birth control hormones) and make them less effective. So be sure to research its drug interactions and check with your healthcare advisor before taking St. John's wort.

Valerian

Valerian root can be helpful for its many calming properties.

BENEFITS

- Reduces anxiety.
- Helps prevent convulsions, seizures.
- Reduces muscle tension.
- Blunts pain.
- Promotes sleepiness.
- May help prevent migraines.

HOW TO USE IT

- Take it (in pill/capsule form or as an herbal tea) 30 minutes to 2 hours before bedtime to help promote sleep.
- The dosage shown most effective in promoting sleep in studies was 450-600 mg. (Higher doses did not appear to offer an increased benefit.)

WHAT YOU NEED TO KNOW

- Valerian acts on the same areas of the brain as certain antidepressant/anti-anxiety drugs and sleep medications, so you should not use valerian if you are taking any of these.
- Unlike many drugs, valerian is not habit-forming.

Low-dose Valium

Although Valium (diazepam) is a prescription anti-anxiety drug, I have included it here to cover one unconventional use: *to prevent or treat true vertigo* (a dizzy/spinning sensation).

HOW TO USE IT

- Take 2-10 mg every 4-6 hours until warning signs stop or the spinning subsides, then wean off.
- Use only for short periods (under 5 days). Prolonged use can prevent natural inner ear healing and stabilization.

Zinc

Zinc is a mineral that is most often associated with a healthy immune system. Many of its benefits can be attributed to simply reversing a zinc deficiency.

BENEFITS

- Promotes healing after injury.
- Boosts immune system.
- Helps prevent macular degeneration of the eyes.
- May improve hearing and reduce tinnitus (ringing in ears) especially with ginkgo biloba.
- Prevents oxidation of other nutrients and vitamins.
- Promotes detoxification through chelation of heavy metals.

HOW TO USE IT

- Approximately 30-50 mg/day should be sufficient. Never exceed about 100 mg/day without a healthcare advisor's guidance.
- May be even more effective when taken with selenium.

19| Vitamin Solutions

In this chapter we will talk about the vitamins you may find helpful for maintaining your youthfulness and vitality. We have included vitamin D here because that's where you'd expect to find it, though it is technically a hormone (or pro-hormone).

Vitamin A (Retinol)

Vitamin A is essential for eye health. It can be obtained from liver, cod liver oil and carrots as well as green leafy vegetables.

BENEFITS

- Promotes healthy vision.
- Supports immune function.
- Increases bone metabolism.
- Improves skin health.
- Serves as an antioxidant.
- May reduce acne.

WHAT YOU NEED TO KNOW

- Vitamin A can be toxic in high doses. Consult your healthcare advisor before supplementing.

B Vitamins

The B vitamin family generally provides energy and reduces inflammation and heart disease.

All B vitamins are water soluble, which means you will pee them out after about 8-12 hours. If your B vitamins come from supplements rather than foods, you may need to take multiple doses each day to maintain steady blood levels.

The B vitamin family includes:
- Vitamin B1 *(thiamine)*
- Vitamin B2 *(riboflavin)*
- Vitamin B3 *(niacin or niacinamide)*
- Vitamin B5 *(pantothenic acid)*
- Vitamin B6 *(pyridoxine, pyridoxal, pyridoxamine, or pyridoxine hydrochloride)*
- Vitamin B7 *(biotin)*
- Vitamin B8 *(inositol)*
- Vitamin B9 *(folic acid)*
- Vitamin B12 *(various cobalamins; typically cyanocobalamin and methylcobalamin in vitamin supplements)*

OVERALL BENEFITS

The B vitamins provide a number of general benefits:
- Support healthy metabolism, provide energy.
- Maintain skin and muscle tone.
- Ensure proper nervous system function.
- Support immune system.
- Support adrenal function.
- Promote cell growth, especially of red blood cells; prevent B-deficiency anemia.

WHAT YOU NEED TO KNOW ABOUT B VITAMINS

Many of the B vitamins need at least one other member of the B vitamin family in order to deliver their benefits. For this reason, it makes sense to take a general B-complex supplement along with any specific B vitamins you may also wish to supplement at higher levels.

Each vitamin in this family has its own particular strengths. Most of these benefits come from reversing a deficiency of the given vitamin. If you are getting enough nutrients from your food, you may never need to supplement B vitamins.

THIAMINE (VITAMIN B1)

Thiamine deficiency can affect the nervous system and brain, causing irregular heartbeat, weight loss, bloating and emotional disturbances.

Thiamine is most plentiful in foods such as wheat germ, rice, lentils, peas, lean pork, Brazil nuts, pecans, oranges, and milk.

RIBOFLAVIN (VITAMIN B2)

Riboflavin deficiency can cause sore throat, mouth swelling or cracks around the mouth, tongue redness, cataracts, sensitivity to sunlight, and scaly skin.

Pregnant women who are deficient in B2 may be more susceptible to pre-eclampsia than those who are not.

Riboflavin can be found in enriched cereals, eggs, fish, meat, almonds, spinach and broccoli.

NIACIN (VITAMIN B3)

Niacin (nicotinic acid) helps your body turn carbs into energy. Niacin also helps keep your nervous system, digestive system, skin, hair and eyes healthy.

Niacin is the B vitamin that causes the hot flush many people dislike. However, niacin can be quite helpful, especially to regulate cholesterol levels.

Niacin can be found in foods such as salmon, fortified cereals, chicken and turkey.

If you take niacin supplements, either ramp up slowly from a very low dose or use a non-flushing form of the vitamin.

PANTOTHENIC ACID (VITAMIN B5)

Deficiency of pantothenic acid is extremely rare. Most Americans get more than enough B5 in their diets.

PYRIDOXAMINE (VITAMIN B6)

Vitamin B6 may be known by a number of names: pyridoxine, pyridoxal, pyridoxamine, or pyridoxine hydrochloride. Pyridoxamine is the biologically active form of the vitamin.

Pyridoxamine, in particular, is especially helpful in reducing age-related deterioration. B6 works synergistically with B12 and folate, especially in preventing age-related diseases.

B6 BENEFITS

- Reduces risk of colon cancer.
- Prevents heart disease (reduce inflammation).
- Lowers blood pressure and cholesterol.
- Reduces risk of carpal tunnel syndrome.
- Prevents symptoms of PMS.
- Improves memory, especially in older adults.
- Improves mood.
- Increases vividness and memory of dreams.
- Reduces water retention.
- Relieves morning sickness and hangover.

- Helps remove heavy metals.
- May prevent or slow progression of diabetic neuropathy.

PYRIDOXAMINE AND THE FDA

Pyridoxamine has been the subject of controversy since 2009 when the FDA reclassified this form of B6 as a drug because it is the active ingredient in a patented drug that helps prevent diabetic neuropathy. Many health-conscious citizens have opposed this ruling, which aims to take pyridoxamine off the market as an inexpensive natural supplement.

As of this writing, pyradoxamine supplements are still available and can be helpful in preventing or slowing the progression of neuropathy.

BIOTIN (VITAMIN B7)

Biotin may sometimes be included as part of an adrenal support therapy.

BIOTIN BENEFITS

- Biotin is primarily useful in helping your body regulate blood sugar.
- It may be (incorrectly) referred to as "vitamin H," since it promotes the healthy growth of hair and nails when taken systemically.

WHERE IT COMES FROM

It is produced by the bacteria in your gut, which typically make more than your body needs. However, if your gut bacteria have been killed off by antibiotics (deliberately taken or consumed in meats that contain antibiotics), you may need to add biotin while you are also restoring your gut with probiotics.

DEFICIENCY

Biotin may be depleted in alcoholics, those who have had gastric bypass, those with certain metabolic disorders, diabetics, epileptics, athletes, and pregnant or lactating women.

Signs of biotin deficiency may include:

- Hair loss
- Conjunctivitis (pink eye)
- Dermatitis/scaly rash on the face
- Depression, lethargy, hallucinations
- Numbness of the extremities (neuropathy)

HOW TO GET IT

Unless you are at risk for deficiency, your gut should make plenty of biotin.

Although many foods contain some biotin (egg yolk, liver), if you are deficient, you will probably need to supplement it.

INOSITOL (VITAMIN B8)

Inositol deficiency can be an underlying contributor to a variety of psychological conditions including bulimia, depression, obsessive-compulsive disorder and agoraphobia.

Supplementation with specific forms of inositol has shown effective in treating such psychological conditions and may also reduce some symptoms of polycystic ovary syndrome (PCOS).

B8 is typically most plentiful in fortified foods (breads, cereals).

FOLATE/FOLIC ACID (VITAMIN B9)

Folate can help prevent age-related degeneration of the brain. It has also been shown to reduce heart disease risks.

Folate is the B vitamin that pregnant women are urged to supplement for its ability to prevent neural-tube defects in developing fetuses.

The rest of us may be getting plenty of B9 in our diets. Folate is found in green, leafy vegetables, as well as peas, beans, lentils, live baker's yeast and fortified breads and cereals.

FOLATE/B9 AND B12 TO PREVENT HEART DISEASE

If you are supplementing B12, you should also supplement folate. The combination of B9 and B12 (and B6) reduces levels of homocysteine—an indicator of inflammation—and together they help prevent heart disease.

THE COBALAMINS (VITAMIN B12)

Most of us know that B12 deficiency can lead to persistent fatigue and a very specific type of anemia.

What we probably don't know is that B12 actually refers to a whole family of B12 vitamins known as cobalamins. The common form of B12 that we get in typical B12 supplements is called *cyano*cobalamin.

But just in the past decade a more bio-active form of B12 called *methyl*cobalamin was discovered that protects against neurological deterioration and aging.

METHYLCOBALAMIN (METHYL-B12)

Your liver can make a small amount of this methyl-B12 from the cyano-B12 you supplement or get in foods, but you really need a lot more.

Methyl-B12 is a powerful brain detoxifier. In sufficient quantities, it can prevent the death of brain cells caused by glutamate toxicity. Glutamate is a necessary neurotransmitter, but when it is released in excessive amounts (as caused by excitotoxins like MSG and others in junk food), it literally kills brain cells.

Methyl-B12 can treat or protect against:

- Chronic fatigue immune dysfunction syndrome (CFIDS)
- Fibromyalgia
- Cognitive/neurological deterioration and toxicity
- Multiple sclerosis (visual and auditory symptoms)
- Peripheral neuropathy
- ALS (Lou Gherig's disease)
- Cancer

GENERAL B12 BENEFITS

B12 is important in preventing or treating a number of symptoms or conditions:

- Heart/cardiovascular disease (by reducing inflammation)
- Fatigue
- Brain fog
- Migraine headaches

TESTING VITAMIN B12

A plain old blood count (CBC test) may flag a possible B12 deficiency. If the "MCV" entry on your results is *lower* than normal you may have an iron-deficiency anemia. If the MCV results are *higher* than normal, you may have a B12 deficiency.

HOW TO USE VITAMIN B12 & METHYL-B12

Vitamin B12 is found primarily in eggs and meat and in certain vitamin-fortified foods, but those sources may not be sufficient.

- **Form.** B12 supplements can be found in a number of forms: pills, sublingual (under the tongue) tablets, nasal sprays, and injectables. For those who are severely B12 deficient, your healthcare advisor may recommend B12 shots initially to ramp your levels up quickly, followed by a maintenance regimen of pills or sublinguals.

- **Dose**. To protect against neurological aging, a dose of 1-5 mg per day may suffice, though patients with MS have been given 60 mg daily.

- **Timing.** Because B12 decreases melatonin levels and promotes alertness, it's best to take it in the morning.

- **Take it with** B6 and B9 (folate/folic acid) for optimal benefit.

Vitamin C (Ascorbic Acid)

Vitamin C is a powerful antioxidant. What many don't know is that it is also a virucidal (kills viruses).

BENEFITS

- Reduces inflammation.
- Kills viruses (in high doses, especially when taken with quercetin), can prevent colds, flu.
- Boosts immune system.
- (In high doses, often given intravenously) may reduce the symptoms of fibromyalgia and chronic fatigue syndrome.
- Helps counteract the effects of stress.
- Helps prevents certain cancers.

HOW TO USE IT

- Vitamin C can be taken orally in surprisingly high dosages. A normal daily dose for an average-size female may be 2000 mg or more (4000 mg for larger males) taken either in two doses (1000 mg twice a day) using time-released pills, or in multiple smaller doses at 8-hour intervals throughout the day.

- Be sure to take quercetin with vitamin C to prevent oxidation and to optimize anti-virus benefits.

WHAT YOU NEED TO KNOW

- Vitamin C is a water-soluble vitamin. That means it can process out of your system through the kidneys in about 8 hours. Even time-released products are eliminated after about 12 hours.

- Also, vitamin C is an acid and may upset your stomach or cause diarrhea in extremely high doses.

- To minimize the acid impact and to keep a steady level of vitamin C in your system, look for products that are *time released* or *sustained release* formulations. You will still need to space out your dosage, for example taking half of your daily dose with breakfast and the other half at dinner.

- You can take as much vitamin C as you need, up to "bowel tolerance" dosages (i.e., until you get diarrhea).

- Vitamin C is more effective at *preventing* infections than *fighting* them, so it is best to include vitamin C in your daily regimen.

- Studies have shown that the more your system is compromised by illness, injury or stress, the more vitamin C you can take without experiencing bowel problems (diarrhea).

- If you decide to cut back or quit taking vitamin C, it's best to reduce your dosage in stages over time, otherwise you may temporarily experience some of the symptoms of vitamin C deficiency. The most common symptom is bleeding gums. These symptoms should fade once your vitamin levels have stabilized again at the lower level.

Vitamin D3

When I talk about vitamin D here I am specifically referring to vitamin D3 unless otherwise noted.

BENEFITS

- Helps prevent nearly all cancers.
- Strengthens bones, prevents osteoporosis.
- Helps prevent heart disease, autoimmune diseases, osteoarthritis.
- Normalizes blood pressure, blood sugar and clotting.
- Reduces inflammation.

HOW TO USE IT

- If you get out in the sun on a regular basis without sunscreen or cover-up for 10 minutes or so (more if you have darker skin or are older), you may be making plenty of D3 in your skin. But in the winter, or if you are in an area closer to the poles where days are shorter or the sunlight is indirect and weak, you may need to supplement D3.
- 2000 IU/day or more may be needed to get blood levels—per the 25(OH)D blood test—into the range of 60-80 ng/mL

WHAT YOU NEED TO KNOW

- Unless you get plenty of sunshine, this may be the most important supplement you can take. *(See The Top 2 Secrets for Women in Chapter 1.)*
- Vitamin D3 supplements are safe and very affordable.

Vitamin E

Vitamin E consists of four tocopherols: alpha, beta, gamma and delta. Alpha tocopherol is the most bio-available, but gamma tocopherol may offer the most benefits.

Vitamin E is best known as an antioxidant. It may also help prevent some symptoms of menopause. And it can help prevent hormone-related cancers.

WHAT YOU NEED TO KNOW

- Vitamin E is fat soluble; therefore, a once-daily dosage can provide sustained protection.

- Take vitamin E (gamma tocopherol) 200 mg per day to prevent hormone related cancers.

- You may need to take mixed tocopherols (alpha, beta, gamma, delta) to ensure you are getting the full spectrum.

- Vitamin E has a blood-thinning effect. Consult your healthcare advisor before taking vitamin E if you are taking other blood-thinning supplements or drugs. Quit taking vitamin E one to two weeks before having any surgeries, and only resume taking it when your surgeon okays it.

20 | Hormone Solutions

As you learned in Chapter 14, hormones are those substances produced by various organs and glands in the body and brain that orchestrate virtually every important function in your body.

Hormones work in harmony with one another and depend on each other, in the right proportions, to support their work.

Under optimal circumstances, all those hormone-producing glands and organs go about their business with no need for tinkering. But as we age, or when things go awry, these systems may need help in order to get back in tune.

This section covers some of the hormones whose supplementation may prove especially useful.

HORMONE REPLACEMENT CHOICES: REAL VS. FAKE

Hormone replacement therapy (HRT or simply HT) traditionally refers to the sex hormones, though technically it can refer to the replacement of any hormone, including thyroid, insulin or cortisol.

When you are faced with the need to supplement one hormone or another, you may have many choices. These choices can usually be divided into two types: bio-identical and bio-deviant. Both may activate some or all of the same responses from your cells, but they are different in important ways.

Bio-identical Hormones

Bio-identical hormones are *chemically identical* to the ones nature gave you. That means:

- Your body recognizes them as the same old hormones it's been seeing all your life. It can use them just as efficiently and safely as the ones you were born with.

- Your body's natural enzymes can easily fit their keys into the hormone molecules' keyholes in order to break down the molecules and flush them out after they've turned on (or turned off) the desired actions.

- Any related hormone tests you might take will clearly reflect the levels of the bio-identical hormones you've been supplementing as if they were produced by your own glands.

The term *bio-identical*, as used throughout this book (and across the medical community), refers to a hormone molecule's match to *human* hormones.

Bio-identical hormones may be converted in a lab from plants. Or they may be obtained directly from animals whose hormones happen to be identical to ours.

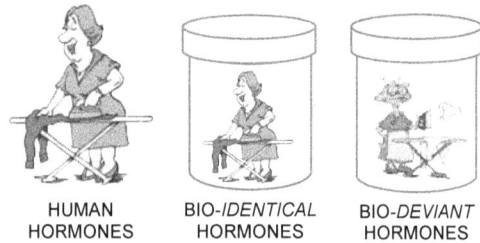

HUMAN HORMONES

BIO-*IDENTICAL* HORMONES

BIO-*DEVIANT* HORMONES

Pig thyroid, for example, contains the same thyroid hormones humans have, in roughly the same proportions. That's why some doctors prefer to use thyroid products obtained from pigs rather than bio-deviant drugs that merely mimic the actions of individual thyroid hormones.

BIO-DEVIANT HORMONES

Horse urine, on the other hand—which is used in certain hormone replacement drugs—contains one bio-*identical* estrogen (estrone/E1) plus several very potent bio-*deviant* horse estrogens.

Studies have found increased disease risks in women using horse-derived and synthetic hormones. But science cannot yet tell us exactly what effects these "alien" hormones have on your organs and on the natural processes within your body over time.

Although bio-deviant hormones—whether from animals, plants or chemicals—are alien to the human body, they may serve useful purposes under certain circumstances.

For example, we do not currently use bio-identical hormones for birth control because the human body processes them too efficiently. Without some means to sustain bio-identical hormone levels consistently throughout the month, we cannot guarantee that a women would not ovulate.

Instead, we use synthetic hormones in contraceptives *precisely because* they are alien and are harder to process out.

However, current research into using progesterone to simulate the conditions of pregnancy in which a woman does not ovulate may eventually lead to the development of an effective bio-identical contraceptive.

THE BIAS AGAINST REPLACEMENT OF SEX HORMONES

You should be aware that within the medical community there is something of a bias against replacing sex hormones.

While doctors are typically quick to replace a patient's missing insulin or thyroid hormones, they may hesitate or refuse to replace the sex hormones—estrogen, progesterone and especially testosterone.

This bias may be blamed on three factors:

- The abuses of steroids among athletes.
- The disturbing results of studies, like the Women's Health Initiative (WHI), of women taking bio-*deviant* hormones.
- Practices and mindsets of times gone by when natural processes such as aging were considered irreversible.

However, abuse of a substance doesn't make that substance bad. Studies of bio-*deviant* hormones tell us *nothing* about the actions of bio-*identical* (and natural human) hormones. And we now have reason to believe that many so-called "age-related" diseases are, in fact, related to declining and imbalanced hormones, and that we can prevent these diseases (and slow other symptoms of aging) by restoring hormones to youthful levels.

HORMONES ARE *NOT* LIKE RECREATIONAL DRUGS

The abuses of testosterone have caused many health practitioners to think of all the sex steroids as "recreational drugs," rather than as the essential hormones they are.

The fact that some people may overuse a substance does not make that substance intrinsically bad or frivolous. You can get high (and ultimately kill yourself) by drinking too much water, even though you would die without water.

Some compare those who seek hormone supplementation to heroine addicts, insisting they crave the "high" these hormones offer. You could similarly say that people who are deprived of air feel a kind of euphoria or high when they are able to breathe again, but that does not make them "air addicts," and you would never dream of withholding air from anyone.

Like air and water, hormones are essential to human life. And like low levels of air and water, low levels of hormones can seriously damage any number of physiological systems. To maintain optimal health, you need optimal levels of the chemicals your body was designed to run on.

HORMONE LEVELS THAT ARE "NORMAL FOR YOUR AGE"

Some healthcare practitioners may insist that it is normal to have low or imbalanced hormones at a certain age. Even lab tests that factor in age will indicate different "normal" levels for young patients and older patients.

Normal in these contexts simply refers to levels of hormones commonly found in an average group of similar people. It says nothing about what levels/balances are *best* for your health and longevity.

Some also insist that because low levels are normal for your age there is no need to replace them. This is like saying that it's normal for your car's gas and oil to run low after a certain number of miles and therefore you should not replace them.

If we treated ourselves at least as well as we treat our cars—by maintaining proper levels and balances of the substances we need—we all could live longer, healthier lives.

CLASSES OF HORMONES

Hormones come in three main varieties, classified according to the materials they are made from. The diagram below shows the classes with examples of the hormones within each.

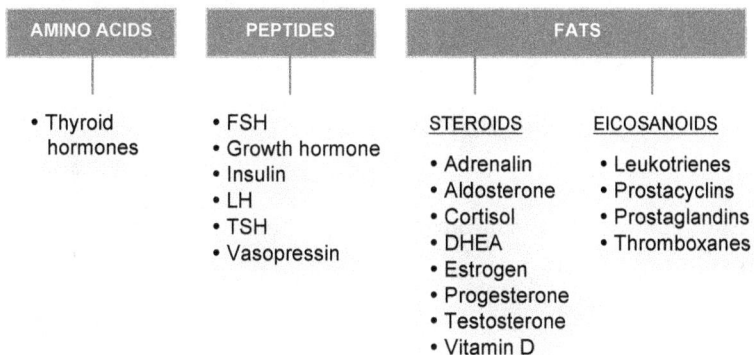

AMINO ACIDS	PEPTIDES	FATS	
• Thyroid hormones	• FSH • Growth hormone • Insulin • LH • TSH • Vasopressin	STEROIDS • Adrenalin • Aldosterone • Cortisol • DHEA • Estrogen • Progesterone • Testosterone • Vitamin D	EICOSANOIDS • Leukotrienes • Prostacyclins • Prostaglandins • Thromboxanes

We will discuss the fat-derived hormones in a bit more detail so you understand where they come from and how you can make them work to your benefit.

STEROIDS (AND STEROLS)

Like most of us, when you hear the word *steroids*, you probably think of bodybuilders and athletes who illegally beef up their muscles with excess hormones, specifically testosterone. That's why steroid hormones have gotten a bad reputation.

However, you should understand that many of the hormones your body needs to function normally are also steroids. Cortisol is a steroid. So is adrenalin, estrogen, progesterone and testosterone. Vitamin D is a closely related sibling in the *sterol* family. And all the steroid/sterol hormones are made from the *master steroid, cholesterol.*

The anti-inflammatory drugs dexamethasone and prednisone are also steroids, but they are *synthetic* steroids, not bio-identical hormones.

All our steroids serve important purposes in making us strong and resilient.

EICOSANOIDS

Most of us have a love/hate relationship with those pesky eicosanoid hormones. We know they're part of an important protective system (the immune system), but we don't like the tools they use to protect us, primarily:

- Pain
- Redness, swelling/inflammation
- Heat/fever

Each of these tools is important to either alert us to a risk or to neutralize a risk.

NSAIDS like aspirin and other pain- and fever-reducing drugs (like COX-2 inhibitors) suppress the production of eicosanoids. These suppressors make you more comfortable and can help limit a fever that might otherwise trigger seizures.

But some doctors believe that by using these drugs too often or too quickly, you may short-circuit the body's natural immune response and may do yourself a disservice in some cases.

For example, if you allow a fever to run its course (as long as it is not dangerously high), your body may more effectively fight off the infection that caused it than if you pop a couple of acetaminophen or ibuprofen pills at the first sign of trouble.

Eicosanoids are made from two very familiar types of fats:

- **Omega-3** essential fatty acids (EFAs) – *suppress* inflammation.
- **Omega-6** essential fatty acids (EFAs) – *promote* inflammation.

The amount and proportions of these fats/oils in your body will influence how your body responds to trauma and disease.

Obviously you need both. Without the inflammation and swelling promoted by omega-6 oils, your body would not be able to heal wounds or create barriers against invading substances or push them out.

But many of us tend to get a lot more omega-6 oils in our diets, especially from fried foods. If those omega-6 oils are not balanced properly with inflammation-suppressing omega-3 oils, you risk overstimulating immune functions until they begin to attack your body for no good reason, increasing allergies and autoimmune diseases and promoting chronic inflammation that can damage your cardiovascular system and joints.

The converse of this is also true. By consuming only omega-3 oils, you may hamper your immune system's ability to respond to disease and damage.

The ideal ratio (depending on which expert you consult) is either an equal balance (1:1) of omega 6 and omega-3 oils, or a 2:1 ratio with twice as much omega-6 as omega-3 oils.

The 4 types of eicosanoids in your immune system's arsenal are:

- **Prostaglandins.** Send pain signals and promote fever.

- **Prostacyclins.** Suppress the formation of blood clots. Dilate (widen) blood vessels. These effects are countered by those of thromboxanes.

- **Thromboxanes.** Constrict (narrow) blood vessels and stimulate the formation of blood clots (to stop bleeding and heal wounds). These effects are countered by those of prostacyclins.

- **Leukotrienes.** Responsible for the inflammation and airway constriction associated with allergies and asthma. They also stimulate the production of mucus.

As you can see, each of the eicosanoids serves a useful purpose, but their effects can be devastating when they are out of control. That's why it is important to maintain a healthy balance of omega-3 and -6 oils.

Even the prostacyclins and thromboxanes counteract one another. This is one more example of the many ways nature uses opposing forces, held in a delicate balance, to keep your body healthy. That's why you need to support those balances through diet and/or supplementation.

ANABOLIC VS. CATABOLIC HORMONES

Hormones (steroids and non-steroids) can be either *anabolic* (tissue building) or *catabolic* (tissue consuming).

- *Anabolic* **hormones like testosterone and progesterone** are well known to build muscle, bone and healthy brain cells.

- *Catabolic* **hormones like cortisol and adrenalin/ epinephrine** break down tissues to release their energy for fuel. Melatonin also has some catabolic effects. The breakdown of fats and proteins is a catabolic process.

Again, the recurring theme here is *balance*.

You need tissue *consuming* hormones to produce energy and replace worn out cells. But you also need tissue *building* hormones to remodel and strengthen your body's structures.

BRAND VS. COMPOUNDED BIO-IDENTICAL HORMONES

Some people think bio-identical hormones can only be obtained through compounding pharmacies. *That's false.* Some also think that compounded hormones are not regulated. *That's false too.*

WHAT YOU NEED TO KNOW

- Many bio-identical hormone products are FDA-approved and mass-produced by drug companies in a fixed set of dosages and forms, and they are available at virtually any drug store in the country.

  - Vivelle Dot (estradiol patch) and Prometrium (progesterone pill) are two of the most commonly prescribed brand-name, bio-identical hormone products.

- Some bio-identical hormones (USP progesterone, primarily) are available in over-the-counter products found online and in health food stores.

- In decades past, virtually all drugs were compounded (mixed from raw ingredients) by qualified pharmacists.

- Today, compounding pharmacies prepare customized, bio-identical hormone products from USP-regulated raw ingredients (USP progesterone, USP estradiol, etc.).

- These ingredients cannot be patented by drug companies because they are made by nature. But their quality, potency and purity are tightly controlled by the FDA and the US Pharmocopeia (USP), an internationally recognized standards-setting organization.

- Compounding pharmacies can customize hormones as well as other drugs.

  - If your needs fall between two standardized amounts, they can mix a custom dosage. Or if you use a combination product, they can change the proportions of one ingredient to another.

  - They can mix a drug/hormone with a different filler or without dyes if you happen to be allergic to something in the brand-name product.

  - If you have trouble getting the full benefits of a drug/hormone from pills, they can mix up a cream or gel that delivers the substance through your skin, or a suppository that gets the substance into your bloodstream through your vagina or rectum.

- Compounding pharmacies are closely regulated by state licensing boards, just like all pharmacies.

- You need a doctor's prescription to obtain compounded hormones.

The bottom line is that while drug companies would like you to believe that compounding is the Wild West of hormone dispensing, in truth, the compounding process is well controlled and audited from a number of perspectives...from the ingredients they use...to the stores and the people who work there. In fact, pharmacists who do compounding may have even *more* credentials than the average pharmacist.

FORMS OF HORMONES

When you supplement hormones, especially with compounded hormones, you may have a number of choices regarding the form of hormone you use. Here's what you need to know about some of them:

- **Pills.** Hormones taken orally must survive your stomach acid and enzymes first, then any breakdown processes that occur in the gut and liver before they make it into your bloodstream. This can alter or diminish the hormones your tissues ultimately receive.

    - Studies have shown that estrogen taken orally increases your risk of blood clots, while estrogen administered transdermally does not increase clotting. (See below.)

- **Transdermals.** Transdermal means *through the skin*. This method gets the hormones directly into your bloodstream without having to pass through the liver first. Transdermal hormones may be in the form of creams/gels or patches.

    - *Creams/gels.* Hormones in this form typically must be applied daily or multiple times a day. Many women will place the hormone on the inside of one wrist and rub it onto the opposite arm. That way, you do not have to lose any of the hormone from washing your hands.

    - *Genital applications.* You may prefer only the genital benefits of hormones like estrogen (lubrication) and testosterone (sexual stimulation) without significantly increasing your overall blood levels of these hormones. If that is the case, you may use the same creams/gels mentioned above, but in smaller doses applied directly to the vagina and/or clitoris.

    - *Patches.* Hormone patches are designed to dispense their hormones a little at time over several days. Some patches are designed to be changed twice a week. Patches are typically applied to flat, hairless areas, like the lower abdomen.

- *Suppositories*. If you like the idea of a transdermal product but have problems with skin irritation or poor permeability of the skin, you can get compounded hormones prepared as suppositories. After insertion, these hormones pass easily through the wall of the vagina or rectum to enter the bloodstream.

- **Sublingual pellets**. Sublingual (under the tongue) hormones are designed to go through the thin tissues under the tongue and directly into the bloodstream. You have to be patient and leave the pellet under your tongue until it has dissolved.

- **Implantable pellets**. Some doctors use hormone pellets that are implanted under your skin every few months. The benefit is that you don't have to worry about taking your hormones every day. But it may take some time and testing to get the dosage right.

- **Injectable hormones**. Currently, the only effective way to administer growth hormone is by injection. These injections are very closely regulated. *We do not recommend using any so-called growth hormone supplements found online.*

WHAT YOU NEED TO KNOW ABOUT HORMONES

- Although age often causes a natural reduction in several hormones, for many of us there may be no compelling reason *not* to correct these deficiencies and imbalances and restore our bodies to optimal health.

- Stress of all kinds can "burn off" certain hormones at a faster than normal rate. For example, a hormone patch that normally lasts 4 or 5 days or more during peaceful times may wear off in only 2 days when you are working around the clock or after you have surgery or an injury.

- Hormones often interact. Supplementing one may enhance or suppress the actions of another. It is important to watch all your key hormones when supplementing any of them.

SPECIFIC HORMONES

The following sections discuss each of the key hormone solutions in detail.

Aldosterone

Aldosterone is a steroid hormone produced in the adrenal glands that helps maintain blood pressure and regulates electrolyte levels.

Declining levels of aldosterone may be a significant cause of age-related loss of hearing. Certain doctors are currently testing bio-identical aldosterone use in patients with hearing loss and vertigo episodes (Meniere's disease).

BENEFITS

- Maintains blood pressure.
- Regulates calcium and potassium levels in the blood.
- Controls processing of fluids through the kidneys.
- May reverse certain types of hearing loss (autoimmune and age-related).
- May prevent or reduce the incidence of vertigo (dizziness).

WHAT YOU NEED TO KNOW

- Aldosterone levels can be measured via blood tests.
- Supplementing aldosterone may increase in blood pressure.
- You may be advised to maintain a low-sodium diet, as sodium can reduce aldosterone levels.

Cortisol, Adrenalin (Epinephrine)

The adrenal glands produce two fuel-delivery hormones: cortisol and adrenalin (sometimes called epinephrine).

Cortisol's job is to provide sustained high levels of energy during times of stress, whereas adrenalin's surge is more intense but short-lived.

CORTISOL

Cortisol's main functions are to help regulate energy levels and to mobilize fuel in response to your body's needs. It is an important part of your immune system, serving as nature's powerful anti-inflammatory hormone...the natural equivalent of drugs like prednisone.

On the negative side, cortisol also counteracts insulin, moves fat deep into your abdomen where it is hard to get out, breaks down collagen in the skin, and destroys cells of all kinds (brain, heart, liver, it doesn't care) in order to liberate fuel to get you through whatever stress you are facing today.

Overall, a high-stress, high-cortisol lifestyle dramatically speeds up the aging process.

Obviously, cortisol is beneficial in the short term to help you survive difficult times. But as mentioned in Chapter 14, you wouldn't choose to routinely burn your furniture to keep your house warm; neither would you want to depend on cortisol to give you energy for normal daily activities.

WHAT YOU NEED TO KNOW

- Excess cortisol can kill brain cells, so it is important to learn how to manage your stress.

- Excess cortisol can eventually burn out your adrenal glands and they will become unable to produce cortisol. *See Adrenal Solutions in Chapter 21.*

ADRENALIN/EPINEPHRINE

Adrenalin is the hormone of panic...and exhilaration. It increases your heart rate, dilates/opens airways and blood vessels and releases a surge of oxygen-rich blood to your brain and muscles in response to emergencies. It also sends a rush of glucose (blood sugar) and fatty acids into your bloodstream.

Adrenalin is the hormone that gives a 98 pound mom the power to lift a 2000 pound car off her child. And it is the hormone that skydivers and other "adrenalin junkies" get high on. It provides a blast of energy resources that quickly burns off.

However, the stresses you face in a given day—being chewed out by the boss, receiving a past-due notice in the mail, even reading an exciting book at bedtime—may provoke surges of adrenalin as well, which can leave you feeling jittery and will keep you up at night.

WHAT YOU NEED TO KNOW

- When you overuse the adrenal glands—through stress or high-risk activities—you run the risk of burning them out. If that happens, you will no longer get that rush of energy, not even in the face of an emergency. *See Adrenaline Therapy in Chapter 21.*

- One way to drain off the excess adrenalin in your system is to enjoy some slow, steady exercise that does not raise your heart rate over 100 beats per minute. Thirty minutes to an hour of walking on a treadmill or 10 minutes of gentle bouncing on a rebounder before bed can help you burn off that remaining adrenalin so you can get a good night's sleep.

DHEA

DHEA is an intermediary hormone best known for its ability to break down into testosterone.

BENEFITS

DHEA provides a number of important functions:

- Breaks down into testosterone.
- Supports memory.
- Builds bone and muscle.
- Normalizes cortisol/adrenalin levels.
- Boosts immune system.
- May reduce appetite, lower body fat.
- Helps normalize cholesterol and blood sugar.

HOW TO USE IT

How you use DHEA depends on the levels you already have in your body and what you want to accomplish with it.

- DHEA levels can be tested effectively via blood or saliva.

- In all cases, you may want to start with a low dose, around 5 mg a day for a week or two, to see how it affects you. Then you can increase dosage to 25 mg or more.

WHAT YOU NEED TO KNOW

- Because DHEA can break down into testosterone, you should watch for symptoms of excess testosterone (facial hair, thinning scalp hair, acne, feelings of aggression, and increased sex drive).

Estrogen

Estrogen is the nurturing, nesting hormone. It makes you put on weight and it calms you, making you less competitive and more cooperative.

Estrogen is the hormone whose deficiency (or sudden withdrawal) is primarily responsible for those hot flashes, night sweats, itchy-crawly feelings, heart palpitations and insomnia associated with menopause.

See Hormonal & Endocrine Processes in Chapter 14, and Menopause Solutions in Chapter 21.

ESTROGEN BENEFITS

- Reduces or relieves classic menopausal symptoms (hot flashes, night sweats, heart palpitations, dry/itchy skin, insomnia, etc.).
- Powerful anti-inflammatory and antioxidant.
- Supports memory and brain function. Decreases risk of Alzheimer's.
- Protects the brain, especially against excitotoxins.
- Reduces the estrogen in the breast and reduces conversion of testosterone into estrogen.
- Slows bone loss.
- Protects against heart disease.
- Reduces/prevents hormone-related incontinence.
- Primes your cells to take in and use progesterone.

THREE ESTROGENS

There are actually 3 key forms of estrogen:

- **E1/estrone** (a moderately strong estrogen) 10%
- **E2/estradiol** (the strongest estrogen) 10%
- **E3/estriol** (the weakest estrogen) 80%

E1/ESTRONE

During reproductive years, estrone (E1) is made in the ovaries. After menopause, it is the dominant form of estrogen, made in fat cells.

E1 is used in a few HRT products (primarily horse-urine-based products). But some believe the E1 made in fat is more prone to stimulate cancers. This may explain why obese women have an increased risk of breast and endometrial cancers.

E2/ESTRADIOL

Estradiol is the primary estrogen in your body. It is also the strongest estrogen. That's why it is the form of bio-identical estrogen most often used for HRT.

The classic symptoms of menopause are thought to be primarily the result of low and or rapidly declining E2 levels. For that reason, E2 is considered the gold-standard for resolving those symptoms unless your risk profile warrants more caution.

E3/ESTRIOL

Estriol is the weakest estrogen and it is typically made from the breakdown of the stronger estrogens E1 and E2.

E3 is considered a protective estrogen and may be used in some compounded bio-identical hormone mixes such as the popular "Bi-est" compound which contains about 20% E2 and 80% E3.

However, E3 may not have the impact on symptoms that E2 can have. You may need either a higher dose of the 20/80 Bi-est, or your doctor may change the proportions, to a 50/50 mixture for example, or may try just E2 alone for a while.

Because E1 and E2 can break down into E3, some doctors will prescribe only E2 initially, then order blood tests to see how much E3 you end up with after that E2 has broken down. We still don't know whether E3 is inherently protective or if it is simply less likely to stimulate cell division because it is weak.

ESTROGENS DURING PREGNANCY

During pregnancy, the strong estrogen, E2, increases 100 times normal levels, while E3, the weak estrogen, increases 1000 times normal. Both are balanced by a 300-times increase in progesterone. These pregnancy hormone levels and proportions appear to protect many birth mothers from getting hormone-related cancers later in life.

THE 2/16 RATIO

As discussed earlier, estrogens can break down in two general directions: one good (the 2 metabolite), the other (the 16 metabolite) more likely to be associated with cancer.

The good news is that you can influence this breakdown process to favor the good metabolite of estrogen by eating certain vegetables (like broccoli). *See The 2/16 Ratio in Chapter 14.*

HOW TO USE IT

- Bio-identical prescription estrogen (E2/estradiol) is available in many forms, including pills, creams and patches. You can find it in brand-name products as well as custom-compounded preparations.

- Your doctor may recommend you use it daily at a consistent dose, or may prefer that you mimic the cycles of nature, ramping up in dosage for two weeks to a peak, then slowly reducing the dosage for the next two weeks.

- Like all topical hormones, estrogen can rub off on clothing, bedding, people and even pets. So take appropriate measures to avoid "sharing." *See Menopause Solutions in Chapter 20.*

WHAT YOU NEED TO KNOW

- Estrogen can be tested effectively using either blood or saliva.

- You need between 35 and 75 times more progesterone than estrogen to offset the potentially harmful effects of estrogen.

- Estrogen delivered transdermally does not increase risk of blood clots, whereas the oral/pill-form can.

- Because estrogen builds glands in the breasts, you may initially experience breast tenderness when starting an estrogen-replacement regimen.

- *See Menopause Solutions in Chapter 21.*

Growth Hormone

Growth hormone may be referred to as GH or as hGH (for *human growth hormone* or bio-identical growth hormone). Our bodies make a lot of it during our formative years, then the levels drop off dramatically beginning around age 30. By age 45, we've lost most of our GH.

BENEFITS

- Improves brain function and mood.
- Increases blood flow to the heart and promotes cardiovascular health.
- Improves lung function.
- Builds bone and muscle, reduces fat.
- Boosts immune function, promotes healing.
- Protects joints and cartilage.
- Supports libido/sex drive.
- Stimulates normal growth in virtually every cell of the body, especially nerve cells.
- Regulates metabolism, burns fats.
- Improves tissue (including skin) elasticity, tightens up sagging jowls, breasts, etc.
- Reduces anxiety.

WHAT YOU NEED TO KNOW

- An IGF-1 blood test can determine your GH levels.
- Some may argue that we no longer need GH after our bodies have matured. But while GH is not needed in those high, developmental levels, it still is essential for maintenance of nearly all physiologic systems.
- You cannot get the right kind of GH supplements over the counter or online. GH must be prescribed by a doctor.
- GH has been shown in some studies to improve insulin sensitivity (making it easier for you to burn off calories). However, other studies have shown just the opposite. In either case, be aware that GH therapy could have an impact (positive or negative) on your metabolism and food cravings.

- GH tends to make your body conserve carbs, so it may be best to reduce your carb intake. And be sure to exercise and eat protein with every meal if you are taking GH.

- If GH is not properly balanced with estrogen, it may cause bloating/water retention.

- Caffeine can reduce GH levels and increase insulin.

- Thyroid hormone balance is important for growth hormone supplementation to be effective.

Insulin

Although discussion of insulin and diabetes is beyond the scope of this book, there are a few things you need to know regarding the interaction of insulin with the hormones covered here.

WHAT YOU NEED TO KNOW

- When you consume food containing sugars (carbs), your body releases insulin to move that sugar (glucose) into cells.

- Glucose is the primary fuel your body is designed to run on every day.

- Insulin effectively "knocks on the doors" of cells in the liver, muscles and fat to get them to take in glucose from the bloodstream to store as potential fuel.

- *Insulin resistance* is a condition in which your body no longer responds properly to insulin. (Insulin is knocking, but the cells don't hear and their doors don't open.)

  - This may be caused by genetic conditions, but more often occurs because your diet is too high in carbs and sugars.

  - This poor response to insulin (cell doors don't open) leaves large amounts of glucose in your bloodstream (high blood sugar), which makes your pancreas release even *more* insulin in an attempt to again try to open those doors and move the sugar into the cells.

- Now you have a lot of insulin in your system.

- Insulin encourages cells to burn carbs before fats. So when you are insulin resistant, those high insulin levels make you crave carbs and make it very difficult for you to burn off fat stores.

- Insulin resistance may be the key reason so many of us have a hard time losing weight.

- If insulin resistance becomes too severe and the pancreas can no longer secrete enough insulin to regulate blood sugar levels, you may be diagnosed with type 2 diabetes. One of the best solutions for this form of diabetes involves dietary changes.

- *See Weight Management Solutions in Chapter 21.*

- Insulin resistance may be one cause of polycystic ovary syndrome (PCOS).

Melatonin

Melatonin is the hormone that helps you get a good night's sleep. But it also has several extremely critical jobs in helping you stay youthful and healthy.

BENEFITS

- Promotes sleep.
- Lowers estrogen production every night.
- Protects heart and cardiovascular system.
- Is one of the most potent anti-inflammatories and antioxidants; boosts immunity, helps prevent/fight cancer, AIDS, ALS, etc.
- Protects the pancreas.
- Regulates body weight, promotes weight loss.

- Reduces symptoms of aging.
- Fights viral and bacterial infections.
- May help improve libido.
- Promotes learning and memory.
- Helps convert cholesterol into bile in the gallbladder.
- May help those with autism and ADHD.
- May help reduce menopausal symptoms, raising prolactin, lowering FSH, supporting thyroid function, reducing depression.
- May prevent headaches (especially cluster and migraine headaches).
- Helps reset your body's internal clock when traveling to and from distant time zones or when changing work shifts.

HOW TO USE IT

- Because ordinary melatonin pills will wear off after about 4 hours, it's best to use a time-released melatonin product or a melatonin patch that slowly releases melatonin into your system over about 6 or more hours.

- The typical dose found in OTC products is 3 mg. However, some people may need up to 20 mg of melatonin to get the restful sleep they need, especially for shift workers who have to sleep during the day.

- Melatonin should typically be taken about 30-60 minutes before your planned bedtime. This helps your body gradually wind down from the day and prepare for sleep.

WHAT YOU NEED TO KNOW

- Melatonin is produced in the pineal gland of your brain when it senses darkness. It is also produced in the retina (eye) and in the gut.

- Melatonin works best when you have enough calcium in your system.

- Melatonin suppresses estrogen production, so if you are not getting enough estrogen, taking melatonin may cause you to wake during the night with hot flashes and other symptoms.

Pregnenolone

Pregnenolone (*preg-NEN-alone*) is the mother hormone, just one step down from cholesterol. Cholesterol breaks down into pregnenolone. All other steroids (sex hormones and the corticosteroids cortisol and adrenalin) come from the breakdown of pregnenolone.

BENEFITS

- Breaks down into progesterone, testosterone, and estrogen, or into cortisol/adrenalin.
- Powerful brain booster (100 times stronger than DHEA).
- Helps increase energy.
- Reduces depression.
- Protects joints, may relieve symptoms of rheumatoid arthritis.
- Promotes healing.

HOW TO USE IT

- Pregnenolone is available in over-the-counter supplements and in compounded prescription creams and other products.
- Like all topical hormones, pregnenolone can rub off on clothing, bedding, people and even pets. So take appropriate measures to avoid "sharing." *See Menopause Solutions in Chapter 21.*

WHAT YOU NEED TO KNOW

Because pregnenolone can ultimately break down into estrogens and testosterone through several different pathways, its supplementation may be helpful for women who can't seem to get the desired benefits from more direct HRT methods (i.e., taking estrogen, progesterone or testosterone).

Progesterone

Progesterone is typically thought of as the hormone of pregnancy, but it also performs a great many other critical jobs on a daily basis throughout your life.

Progesterone is important both to balance the effects of estrogen and to deliver the many benefits of the hormone itself.

During reproductive years, your body contains between 35 and 75 times more progesterone than estrogen, depending upon the time of the month (and even more during pregnancy). So if you had 1 teaspoon of estrogen in your system, you also had between 35 and 75 teaspoons of progesterone in your system to prevent the negative effects of runaway estrogen.

As you get older, those proportions shift, with progesterone levels declining far more dramatically than estrogen, until at some point you have too little progesterone to effectively "oppose" estrogen.

When that happens, your body is in a state of *"estrogen dominance,"* which can promote the development of estrogen-sensitive cancers and other diseases.

Even if you don't restore your hormones to youthful *levels*, you should at least reestablish the youthful *proportions* to protect yourself against devastating disease.

BENEFITS

- Helps prevent estrogen-sensitive cancers.
- Eases anxiety/depression.
- Promotes sleep (especially oral progesterone).
- Builds strong bones, muscles.
- Prevents/reduces PMS.
- Calms irregular/heavy periods.
- Supports brain & memory.
- Protects myelin (insulation) for nerves, spinal cord, brain, and calms central nervous system.
- Increases metabolism, decreases appetite, promotes weight loss.
- Decreases water weight, bloating.
- Supports heart/cardio health, normalizes cholesterol.
- Promotes sex drive/libido.
- Reduces/normalizes blood clotting.
- Reduces allergies.
- Normalizes blood sugar.

See Introduction for more information.

HOW TO USE IT

- A blood or saliva hormone test will tell you: (a) how low your progesterone is, and (b) how low it is relative to your estrogen levels.
- Your first goal should be to reestablish the normal proportions (between 1 to 35 and 1 to 75) of E to P
- Replacing progesterone can be quite easy with the many over-the-counter creams and gels on the market. Just make sure the ingredients include "USP progesterone" (bio-identical).

- You may also get progesterone by prescription, whether compounded or in brand-name products.

- You can take the same dose every day, or your doctor may prefer that you mimic nature by using a low dose daily (or none) for two weeks of each month, then ramping up to a higher dose for the remaining two weeks. *See Menopause Solutions in Chapter 21.*

- Your body fat may "stockpile" some of the progesterone you've administered as a topical cream. If that happens, you may think you are getting too little at first, then, as you continue to take regular doses *and* those stockpiles begin to release some of that stored progesterone, you may end up with too much in your system.

- It's best to start slow, giving your body time to adjust, and test progesterone levels at least 4 to 6 weeks following each significant change in your regimen.

- Like all topical hormones, progesterone can rub off on clothing, bedding, people and even pets. So take appropriate measures to avoid "sharing."

WHAT YOU NEED TO KNOW

- Many studies have proven the safety and effectiveness of bio-identical progesterone.

  - For example: In the E3N study (Fournier 2005) of 54,000 French women taking some form of progesterone, those using bio-identical progesterone had a *10% lower risk of breast cancer* than average women taking no progesterone, while those taking synthetic (bio-deviant) progesterone had a *40% increase* in the incidence of breast cancer.

- Some women may actually be allergic to their own progesterone. Most doctors are unaware of this. *(See Hormone Allergies in Chapter 17, and Dr. Jonathan Wright information in Chapter 22.)*

- Progesterone and thyroid hormones are closely linked. Many symptoms of low progesterone mirror those of low thyroid. If you suspect problems with one or the other, you should test for both. And if you supplement one, give your body time to react to it fully (at least 4-6 weeks) before you consider testing and supplementing the other.

- *See also: Top 2 Secrets in Chapter 1, and Menopause Solutions in Chapter 21.*

Testosterone

Testosterone is famously (or *in*famously) known for building muscles, promoting aggressive behavior, deepening the voice and growing beards. It is true that testosterone is the hormone that drives all those traditionally "masculine" characteristics. But testosterone is equally important for women.

About half of your testosterone is made in the ovaries; the other half is made in the adrenal glands. If your ovaries are not functioning properly or have been removed, your testosterone levels may drop by 50%...or even more, depending on your enzyme levels.

- **Conversion (aromatization) of testosterone to estrogen.** Your body fat makes an enzyme called *aromatase* that converts testosterone (and its precursor, androstenedione) into estrogens (E2 and E1, respectively). As you get older, you may make more aromatase, causing even more of your testosterone supplies to convert into estrogen.

BENEFITS

Testosterone is critical for strength, endurance, and emotional wellbeing.

It is clearly associated with cardiovascular health. In fact, the heart has more testosterone receptors than any other organ or muscle in the body.

And testosterone is essential for brain health and cognitive fitness. Numerous studies in men have shown that testosterone levels are lowest in those with Alzheimer's, and that both low testosterone and estrogen levels reliably *predict* men who will later suffer from the disease.

Testosterone supplementation offers a variety of important benefits:

- Supports brain function.
- Promotes feelings of wellbeing.
- Builds strong new bone and muscle tissue.
- Decreases risk of breast cancer, heart disease, Alzheimer's.
- Decreases inflammation.
- Normalizes cholesterol levels and blood sugar.
- Promotes sexual desire and fantasy.
- May reverse hormone-related dry eye.

HOW TO USE IT

- Your doctor may prescribe a compounded testosterone formulation that is just right for your needs, provided as a cream in a syringe or in a metered dispenser (which you twist like a lipstick to release the specified dose).

- However, you may be given a prepackaged gel or cream that is designed for men. That means you will have to use only a small fraction (about 1/10th) of the dose recommended for men.

  - If the testosterone is provided in single-dose packets (like fast-food catsup packets), you may have to find a small reclosable container (like an empty lipgloss jar) to keep this intended single dose of gel in while you dip a finger into it and rub a little on your skin each day.

- Like all topical hormones, testosterone can rub off on clothing, bedding, people and even pets. So take appropriate measures to avoid "sharing." *See Menopause Solutions in Chapter 20.*

- If you have high aromatase enzyme levels, you may need to take an aromatase inhibitor to hold onto whatever testosterone you are taking or making naturally. Zinc is a weak aromatase inhibitor and can help a bit, but some people need a drug to fully curb that conversion.

WHAT YOU NEED TO KNOW

- Bio-identical testosterone products for women have been blocked from FDA approval over the past 10 years by people who insist they objectify women or address a need that doesn't really exist except to make money for drug companies. In fact, many women need testosterone supplementation and must rely on cutting down dosages of male-targeted products.

- Instead of supplementing, some women may actually need to *reduce* testosterone or *balance* it with estrogen. Too much testosterone can cause a number of side effects including:
  - Aggressive behavior
  - Acne, oily skin
  - Male-pattern baldness/hair loss; facial hair growth
  - Deepening voice
  - Increased sex drive

Thyroid

An in-depth discussion of thyroid solutions is beyond the scope of the current book. However, one point is relevant to the use of the hormonal solutions covered here and bears repeating.

WHAT YOU NEED TO KNOW

- Progesterone and thyroid hormones influence one another. If you test or supplement one, you should also test and monitor the other.

- *See thyroid discussions under Progesterone section of this chapter. See also Chapter 14: Hormonal and Endocrine Processes.*

21 | Solution Protocols

Some solutions work so well together toward a common purpose that it is worth repeating a few in order to cover their combined ability to prevent or reverse some of the most destructive conditions we face.

Adrenal Therapy

When your adrenals are compromised or burned out, you feel it inside, especially in your low energy levels and susceptibility to disease. But you can also see it on the outside.

When you restore adrenal function, you can also:

- Reduce dark circles under your eyes and age spots on your skin.
- Eliminate edema (fluid/swelling in your tissues).
- Improve flow of lymph, decrease constipation, and increase your excretion of toxins and wastes.
- Increase mental function and concentration.
- Prevent or reduce episodes of dizziness.
- Improve sleep.

Adrenal therapy can include a number of solutions, including:

- **Progesterone and/or its precursor, pregnenolone.** (To help take some of the burden off the adrenal glands, especially while they are recovering from fatigue/exhaustion.)
- **DHEA.** (Because stress depletes DHEA).
- **Vitamin D3.** (Highest concentration of vitamin D in the body is in the adrenals).

- High doses of B vitamins, especially B5/pantothenic acid 500 mg/day, or licorice tea (not recommended for those with high blood pressure), B1, B6.

- High-dose vitamin C.

- Cortisol supplements (if low), phosphatidyl serine and Relora (if cortisol is high).

- CoQ10.

- Possibly carnosine.

- Cut out diet soda and other toxins, improve diet.

- Supplement minerals.

Antioxidants

You may hear people say that cholesterol or omega-6 oils are bad for you. But neither is inherently bad. The problem only comes when they *oxidize*, because oxidized substances can lead to cancer, heart disease and other conditions.

Oxidation is a chemical conversion process similar to what happens when iron rusts. Both require the presence of *oxygen*.

But a lot of very beneficial substances can oxidize, including the powerful *anti*oxidant, vitamin C! Yes, it seems contradictory. But it all goes back to that recurring theme: *balance*.

Just as a car needs an accelerator and a brake, our bodies need well-balanced opposing forces to maintain optimal health.

If we tried to keep everything that can oxidize out of our bodies, we'd die, because many of those substances—like cholesterol, omega-6 oils, and vitamin C—are essential to our health.

The answer is not to avoid these substances, but to nourish our bodies with a *variety* of antioxidants.

MOST POWERFUL ANTIOXIDANTS

While many substances work as antioxidants to prevent the damage caused by free radicals, a side effect of the oxygen we need, a few stand out as the most important:

- Melatonin (one of the few antioxidants that can get past the blood-brain barrier)
- Vitamin C (ascorbic acid)
- Vitamin D3
- CoQ10 (50 times more potent than vitamin E)
- Omega-3 oils (fish, flax, etc.)
- Estrogen
- Glutathione
- Vitamin E (gamma tocopherol or mixed tocopherols)

Bone Therapy

Healthy bones are constantly undergoing a rebuilding, or *remodeling*, process. Every day, old bone cells break down and are replaced by strong new bone cells. And as in every other part of your body, balance is important to keep these two processes equalized.

Building and maintaining strong bones requires four things:

1. **Bone-building materials** (calcium, magnesium, vitamin D, protein, etc.)

2. **Bone-remodeling hormones** (progesterone, testosterone and growth hormone for bone building; estrogen to slow bone loss)

3. **Weight-bearing exercise** (to make existing bone stronger, more dense)

4. **Neutral pH** (to keep your body from pulling calcium out of your bones)

BONE-BUILDING MATERIALS

You need a variety of raw materials to help build bone. Many of these are readily available in your diet, so there is no need to supplement them. Those you may need to be aware of are:

- **Calcium.** The workhorse of bone building, calcium is present in many foods, especially dairy products and vegetables. If you eat a healthy diet, you may not need to supplement calcium. If you do take calcium, it is important that you also supplement magnesium and vitamin D.

  - Be aware that too much calcium can cause joint pain and can change your body's pH balance, which can actually *accelerate bone loss. (See "Neutralize pH" below.)*

- **Magnesium.** Promotes hardness in bones and teeth. You need magnesium in order to use vitamin D and calcium. Without sufficient magnesium, you may develop kidney stones or calcium deposits in your joints. For bone health, magnesium and vitamin D supplementation may be more important than calcium supplementation.

- **Chromium.** Promotes the production of collagen in bone-building cells and slows the rate of normal bone breakdown. *(See also the Weight Loss Solutions section.)*

- **Zinc.** Provides the scaffolding upon which collagen is grown to make bone. Zinc is also important for immune function.

- **Manganese.** Critical for the formation of bone cartilage and collagen as well as bone mineralization.

- **Copper.** Helps strengthen collagen in bone and connective tissues, slows bone loss. Diets high in sugar and flour deplete copper supplies in the body.

- **Potassium.** Neutralizes bone-robbing acids and slows the rate of calcium loss. You can find it in potatoes and bananas.

- **Vitamin D3.** Although many vitamins are important for bone health, none is more important than vitamin D3, which promotes the absorption of calcium from the intestines and kidneys and moves it into the blood.

BONE-REMODELING HORMONES

Bone remodeling requires a controlled amount of *bone loss* and *bone building*. Your sex hormones regulate both these processes.

- **Estrogen.** Slows the rate of bone loss.
- **Progesterone, testosterone, growth hormone.** Build strong new bone.

Most osteoporosis drugs mimic the action of estrogen, that is, they slow the rate of bone loss. By addressing only the bone loss part of the equation, these drugs merely *preserve old bone, without building strong new bone.*

WEIGHT-BEARING EXERCISE

Any form of movement that forces your body to resist the pull of gravity (or any opposing force) will increase bone density and strength. Even walking or doing housework can be considered weight-bearing exercise. If you add weights, you will get even more bone benefits.

NEUTRALIZE PH

Your body prefers to be in an essentially neutral pH state, just slightly toward the alkaline (base) side.

When your blood is too acidic, your body does exactly what you do when you think your stomach is too acidic: it adds calcium to neutralize it. But where does it get that calcium? It steals it from your bones and muscles.

So to maintain healthy bones and muscles, you want to avoid excess acid in your system. To do this you need to balance the proteins and meats you eat (which break down into acids) with citrus fruits (which break down into bases).

Although you can neutralize acidic pH with calcium tablets or baking soda, these can neutralize the stomach acid you need to break down your food, so it's best to focus on dietary solutions.

Brain and Mood Solutions

As your body changes, you may find that your moods change, and your ability to remember or process information declines. But these changes may not be inevitable.

Hormones and other supplements can help reverse or prevent many of these unwelcome effects.

HORMONES

- **Pregnenolone**, the mother hormone from which all the sex hormones are made, has a powerful memory-enhancing effect on the brain.

- **Estrogen** is known for its mood-stabilizing benefits; it is the hormone of nurturing and nesting. It also promotes brain health. Studies of women who have had their ovaries removed have shown that estrogen supplementation is essential to restoring or maintaining memory and cognitive function after estrogen-impacting surgery.

- **Progesterone** has a gentle mood-elevating and anti-anxiety effect and it is critical for proper brain function. Virtually every kind of brain cell contains progesterone receptors. Taken orally in the evening, progesterone may also help some women fall asleep.

- **Testosterone** is the classic feel-good hormone. It promotes overall feelings of wellbeing, and also drives healthy sexual fantasies and desires. Testosterone is critical for healthy brain function and memory.

SUPPLEMENTS

- **SAMe.** A natural antidepressant. Well known among midwives for its ability to relieve post-partum depression faster and with fewer side effects than conventional antidepressants.

- **St. John's Wort.** An antidepressant herb shown in studies to reduce depression as effectively as conventional antidepressants with fewer side effects.

- **Omega-3 oils.** Supplementing omega-3 oils can reduce depression and improve memory.

- **Folic acid (folate).** Studies of people over 50 have shown that supplementing folic acid/folate dramatically increases cognitive function.

- **Magnesium.** Improves learning and memory. Effects may be most pronounced when restoring optimal levels in those who have been deficient in magnesium.

- **Phosphatidyl serine (PS).** An essential fatty acid (EFA) found in the membranes of brain cells. Reduces cortisol and supports memory and cognition.

- **Acetyl-l-carnitine (ALC).** Improves brain function, stress tolerance and metabolism. Protects and regenerates nerve cells. Increases the neurotransmitters serotonin and dopamine to help reduce depression. ALC also helps your brain metabolize fat and cholesterol and may help prevent Alzheimer's.

- **Ginkgo biloba.** Although this herb is touted for its memory-enhancing effects, research in this area is inconclusive.

- **N-acetylcysteine, rhodiola rosea, histidine, methionine.** These may be helpful when you need to *stimulate* your overall nervous system.

- **5-HTP, taurine**. These can help *calm* your nervous system.

Cancer Preventive/Fighting Solutions

Preventing and fighting cancer is one of society's biggest challenges, and this section certainly cannot begin to cover all possible solutions. What we offer here are a few of the most effective substances that you may consider adding to your overall health regimen if you are concerned about cancer.

- **Vitamin D3**. Helps prevent nearly all types of cancer.
- **CoQ10**. Has been shown to prevent the recurrence of breast cancer.
- **Curcumin**. Shown to help prevent/fight colon cancer.
- **Indol-3 carbinol (I3C)** (Found in cruciferous vegetables like broccoli, cauliflower, cabbage, Brussels sprouts). Promotes the favorable breakdown of estrogen (the 2/16 ratio), reducing hormone-sensitive cancer risk.
- **Melatonin**. Low melatonin levels are associated with an increased risk of cancer, which suggests that supplementing melatonin may reduce that risk.
- **Selenium**. May help reduce risk of cancer.
- **Lycopene**. Found primarily in tomatoes. Has been found to reduce the risk of many cancers.
- **Cimetidine (Tagamet)**. Initially marketed for heartburn, it didn't work very well. However, it has proven to be quite effective in slowing the progression of colon cancer and other types of cancer.

Chiropractic Solutions

Because your nerves facilitate communications across all parts of your body and your brain, it only makes sense that when your spine is misaligned, those communications can be disrupted.

Chiropractic solutions focus on freeing these communication pathways by restoring proper alignment and relieving pressure on vertebrae and nerves.

Chiropractic solutions can solve a wide range of seemingly unrelated problems, from allergies to limb or back pain, all by restoring the body's normal communications channels.

Dental Solutions

Beyond the obvious benefits, dental treatment can impact other areas of your health, most importantly:

- **Heart health.** Because chronic gum disease and periodontal infection can provoke inflammation — which damages the cardiovascular system — you may be able to prevent heart disease merely by flossing and getting regular teeth cleanings. If you have an infection in the gums or teeth, it can be treated with surgery and/or antibiotics.

- **Headaches.** Many headaches may be related to inflammation from gum/tooth disease or misalignment of the temporomandibular joint (TMJ) at the hinge of your jaw just below the ear. Your dentist can help resolve these headache causes.

Detoxification Solutions

Detoxifying your body involves two processes: getting bad things out and putting good things in. There are a number of ways to do both. The best solution depends on the type of toxicity you have.

GENERAL DETOXIFICATION

INTERNAL CLEANSING

Cleansing may often be your first line of defense when you simply can't keep all toxins out of your body, including yeast (Candida), parasites and neurotoxins from prepared foods.

A typical cleansing routine includes four primary elements:

- Fiber to scrub your GI tract.
- A natural laxative to stimulate your gut.
- Supplements to replace essential vitamins, minerals, etc., that may be lost in the purge.
- Candida troche to suppress yeast overgrowth.

RESTORATIVE SUPPLEMENTS

Supplements that may be most helpful in restoring your immune and detoxification systems to optimal performance after any struggle with toxins include:

- Methylcobalamin, a form of vitamin B12
- Zinc
- Selenium
- Glutathione
- Carnosine

LIVER DETOX

Among the most helpful liver detox or support solutions are:

- Juice of a fresh lemon in 6 oz of water every morning (to flush the liver)
- Milk thistle/silymarin
- Bupleurum

LYMPHATIC DETOX

Sometimes your lymphatic system needs a little help, especially if you don't move around much or have been dealing with a lot of illness or toxicity. Some beneficial (and enjoyable) techniques are:

- **Lymphatic massage.** Any kind of massage will help release some toxins. But an experienced therapeutic massage practitioner knows how to gently "milk" the lymphatic channels and facilitate the drainage of their contents into the bloodstream. You can even do it yourself with some training. The important thing is to know how and where to stroke the skin.
- **Dry brushing.** Another way to stimulate movement in the lymphatic system is to use a soft, dry brush to gently stroke the skin, moving in a specific direction that encourages the lymph to drain.
- **Infrared sauna.** This method gets at the stubborn toxins stored in fat perhaps better than any other method because it allows you to comfortably heat your body longer.

CHELATION AND HEAVY METAL DETOX

Chelation is a process in which you are given a substance that flows through your bloodstream and binds/sticks to heavy metal toxins (lead, mercury, aluminum, iron, cadmium, arsenic, uranium/plutonium, etc.) and helps your body eliminate them.

Other substances helpful when detoxifying your body of heavy metals are:

- Zinc
- Selenium
- Glutathione
- Carnosine

YEAST DETOX

Yeast/Candida normally lives in the human gut without causing any harm. But if you have been sick or your immune system is compromised, yeast can grow out of control, causing various problems including:

- Vaginal yeast infections
- Thrush (yeast overgrowth in the mouth)
- Fatigue or weight gain

REMOVING/REBALANCING YEAST

You can help rebalance your GI tract by laying off sugar and other refined starches and all yeasts for a month or more. This can force you to eat healthier foods in general, which will help reduce your symptoms as well.

If you have been ill, and especially if you've been taking antibiotics, you may also need to add probiotics (friendly gut bacteria), either as pills or in yogurt, for at least two weeks.

If you continue to have digestive problems, you may actually have undiagnosed food sensitivities and should considering having an IgG test.

REVERSING EXCITOTOXIN DAMAGE

Because it is so difficult to eliminate all excitotoxins from your food, it's important know how to remove them from your body and/or repair the damage they can cause. Some of the solutions that can be most helpful include:

- Fish oil (especially the DHA in fish oils)
- B vitamins (especially B12, folate, thiamine, B6, and niacinamide)
- Selenium
- Magnesium

- DHEA
- Glutathione

Dry Eye Solutions

Your eyes are kept moist with tears, which are made up of water, oil and mucus. When those three substances aren't balanced, or when your eyes simply don't make enough tears, your eyes can dry out.

There are a few solutions that may help reverse this condition.

- **Testosterone, DHEA**. Because the layer of oil in tears (as well as your body's overall oil production) decreases as your so-called male hormones decline, many have found that supplementing these hormones can reduce eye dryness. You may be able to find testosterone products (especially compounded) formulated specifically for use in the eyes.

- **Punctal plugs.** In some cases, your doctor can insert tiny plugs into your tear ducts to keep the tears you do make and stop them from draining away.

- **Drugs**. For severe dry eyes, prescriptions such as Restasis may help.

Food Allergy/Sensitivity Solutions

Once you have determined (through testing) that you have a food sensitivity, you can choose to eliminate the bothersome foods from your diet, or you can use a rotation diet to keep them on your plate without suffering the consequences.

ROTATION DIET

The rotation diet involves eating any foods you like from a specific family of bothersome foods on the same day, then avoiding all foods from that family for four or more days before eating them again. This may help keep your immune system from overreacting when you do eat those foods you love that don't love you back.

Remember that if you have leaky gut syndrome as a result of food sensitivities, antigens can pass through your gut into your bloodstream and trigger undesirable immune responses including inflammation.

Incontinence Solutions

As hormones decline, you lose muscle tone and skin elasticity. These changes can manifest in incontinence, or leaking urine.

There are two types of incontinence:

- **Stress incontinence** (You leak urine when you sneeze, laugh, cough or exercise.)

- **Urge incontinence** (You feel an uncontrollable urge to pee at odd times for no apparent reason; sometimes called "overactive bladder.")

Many women have both. A specialist in gynecologic urology can conduct tests and help you decide on the right solutions for you.

STRESS INCONTINENCE

Stress incontinence is related to the lack of tone in the muscles that close off the urethra and to the sagging of your internal organs over time. If you have had a hysterectomy this sagging may be exaggerated.

A few solutions can help manage or relieve this part of the problem:

- **Hormone replacement therapy**. Because the decline in elasticity and muscle tone is related to the reduction in hormones, replacing those hormones can help. Hormones that promote elasticity and muscle tone are progesterone, testosterone, DHEA and growth hormone.

- **Kegel and other exercises**. For some women, learning and practicing these exercises that work the pelvic floor muscles may strengthen these muscles and reduce stress incontinence. Your urologist's team can teach you these techniques.

- **Pads**. If the problem is relatively mild, you may be able to manage it by wearing incontinence pads.

- **Bladder/ureter suspension surgery**. If incontinence is a serious disruption to your life, the urologist can perform a simple and quick (less than 30 minute) surgery called a *slingplasty*. Essentially, the doctor pokes three tiny holes in your pelvic area and installs a thin ribbon that acts like an internal hammock for your ureter to rest on.

URGE INCONTINENCE (OVERACTIVE BLADDER)

While stress incontinence is a *mechanical* issue (lost muscle tone), urge incontinence is a *nerve* issue in which the bladder repeatedly spasms, causing that uncontrollable urge to pee.

The solutions listed above for stress incontinence can help reduce or manage overall leakage, but the bladder spasms of urge incontinence may require additional approaches.

To address the spasms of urge incontinence, the following solutions may be effective:

- **Biofeedback**. Your doctor's team can teach you how to listen to your body's signals and slowly retrain them.

- **Drugs**. Most of the drugs used for controlling overactive bladder have undesirable side effects. Be sure to investigate these before you consider trying one of these drugs.

- **Electrical stimulation** (*external*). Several methods of electrical stimulation pulse the nerves in the pelvic region to contract the muscles of the bladder, urethra and/or vagina in an effort to retrain them.

- **Electrical stimulation** (*internal*). Doctors can implant a tiny electrical device, like a heart pacemaker, attached to the sacral nerve in your pelvis to reset the normal signals to your bladder.

Inflammation Solutions

Reducing inflammation is an extremely important part of any wellness and rejuvenation program. Inflammation creates wrinkles, it damages your cardiovascular system, and it stresses your adrenals and immune system.

TESTING FOR INFLAMMATION

Your healthcare advisor can test your key indicators of inflammation—C-reactive protein (CRP) and homocysteine—via simple blood tests.

And you may also want to test for fasting insulin, since chronic inflammation may increase your risk of type 2 diabetes.

INFLAMMATION AND HEART DISEASE

Inflammation can be caused by any number of things, even recurrent sinus infections or untreated gum disease. You may not even be aware of the cause of the inflammation.

In fact, researchers only discovered the important connection between inflammation and heart disease when they noticed that subjects in their decades-long studies had fewer heart attacks during the winter.

They discovered that in the winter more people had colds and went to their doctors, who then prescribed antibiotics. Those antibiotics (which were useless against the virus that causes the common cold) may have accidentally been treating low-grade infections the patients didn't know they had. And in doing so, the treatment reduced inflammation, which reduced their risk of heart attack.

So it is important to identify and treat *any* infections you may have, and to reduce overall inflammation.

INFLAMMATION SOLUTIONS

Because many of the solutions that fight inflammation also serve in other capacities, we will merely list them here. If they have other benefits, we will discuss those under other sections.

Some of the most important anti-inflammatory solutions are:

- Omega-3 oils (fish, flax, etc.) (higher doses for joint pain and heart disease available by prescription)
- Balanced blood sugar
- Balanced, optimal levels of hormones (esp. progesterone)
- Vitamin D3
- Resveratrol
- Curcumin
- Quercetin and ellagic acid
- CoQ10/ubiquinol
- Milk thistle
- Echinacea

Longevity Solutions

Certainly no discussion of health secrets would be complete without covering the ultimate objective: longer life.

People have been looking for the Fountain of Youth since long before Ponce de León set sail for Florida in the 16th century. But now, science has found a way to extend a person's life span by lengthening or preserving the *telomeres* at the ends of chromosomes.

TELOMERES

Telomeres are bits of DNA that protect the ends of chromosomes like the tips on the ends of shoelaces. Normally, a given cell can only divide a certain number of times because each division shortens its telomeres.

Imagine that telomeres are match heads. If you were stranded in the woods with only one match, you could make two or more matches by splitting the first match. The problem is that at some point you will have divided up the match head into such small portions that it can no longer start a fire. That's similar to what happens with the telomeres each time your cells divide.

The cells in our bodies replace themselves (by dividing to create new cells so the old ones can die) about every 120 days. Cells are programmed for a specific number of divisions (regulated by the length of the telomeres). Once they've reached that number, they can no longer grow or replace themselves with fresh new versions.

When the telomeres are too short to support more divisions, those cells (and the organs they make up) begin to age. That's when we start to see wrinkles, sagging skin and age spots.

What we don't see are the aging processes taking place *inside* our bodies, though we may notice evidence of those processes as we begin to snore at night, or leak urine, or start to develop health problems...because our tissues are no longer rejuvenating themselves.

INCREASING/PRESERVING TELOMERE LENGTH

There are very few solutions currently known that can increase the life span of our cells and they include: calorie restriction, long-term fitness/training, and taking resveratrol.

These methods all work by accomplishing the same thing: they turn our cells back on so they can continue dividing and repairing themselves.

CALORIE RESTRICTION (CR)

Studies in mice have shown that reducing calorie intake by 10% to 25% (the equivalent of consuming under about 1300 calories a day for an average size woman) can significantly increase life span.

Although humans practicing CR have not yet *proven* the life extension benefits of CR (because we don't know how long they ultimately will live), the practice improves any number of factors that contribute to aging (including cholesterol, blood pressure and insulin sensitivity)...and has proven to increase the length of telomeres.

CR can also be practiced by fasting every other day.

RESVERATROL

As it turns out, the miracle substance in red wine that seems to protect the French and Italians from their rich Mediterranean diets also protects the telomeres on the ends of your chromosomes...just like calorie restriction does. *(See the Resveratrol discussion in Chapter18.)*

Science is currently investigating other natural substances in the quest to find more solutions that have anti-aging properties.

LONG-TERM EXERCISE/TRAINING

Latest research indicates that regular vigorous exercise, especially when it is sustained over many years, helps lengthen those telomeres that keep you from aging. Working up a sweat exercising even 3 times every week can add nearly 10 years to your life!

Menopause Solutions

Although menopausal problems can cover a lot of territory, there are a few key solutions that warrant discussion as a protocol. Refer to the relevant earlier sections for details about each solution shown here.

HORMONES

Keep in mind that there is a lot more going on in menopause than the obvious symptoms. Many women think that if they don't have hot flashes there is no need to consider taking hormones.

The truth is that our bodies require the full range of hormones to function optimally. Without them in the proper levels and proportions, we may allow a variety of silent degenerative processes to age us prematurely and rob us of life's pleasures.

The key hormones you may need as you transition out of reproductive mode are:

- **Progesterone.** The first hormone you are likely to need is progesterone. Even during reproductive years, progesterone can help reduce PMS and stabilize your cycles. Later on, progesterone becomes more important to help balance estrogen and to restore brain, bone and muscle health, lift your spirits and prevent hormone-related cancers, heart disease and autoimmune conditions.

- **Estrogen**. For hot flashes, night sweats, heart palpitations, itchy skin, vaginal dryness, and insomnia, no other solution can hold a candle to estrogen, specifically estradiol/E2. It also promotes heart health by normalizing cholesterol and it mellows your mood.

- **Testosterone**. For those who need it, testosterone can be a lifesaver. It can restore your sex drive/libido, reverse depression and brighten your mood, build strong bones and muscles, suppress your appetite, increase lean body mass, sharpen your brain, and reduce the risk of heart disease and hormone-related cancers.

- **Pregnenolone**. The mother hormone from which the other sex hormones are made can provide a different route by which you can improve your memory and increase the benefits of the other hormones.

- **DHEA**. An important part of adrenal therapy, DHEA can improve the adrenal glands' ability to produce those backup supplies of estrogen, testosterone, and tiny bit of progesterone. DHEA can also break down into testosterone.

- **Melatonin**. For insomnia, the best solution is estrogen. But if you can't supplement estrogen, melatonin is the next best option. Be sure to get time-released products and start with 3 mg, increasing dosage every week or so, if necessary, until you get the results you need.

- **Growth hormone**. Because of the controversy around it, GH may be a long shot for most women. But if you test low in GH, supplementing it as part of an overall HRT regimen can literally transform your body and mind, turning back the clock on aging.

WHAT YOU NEED TO KNOW

- Topical hormone creams and gels can rub off on clothing, bedding, people and even pets.

  - Choose your application sites carefully to make sure these areas will not be exposed outside your clothing.

  - Apply to hairless areas like wrists and inner arms, belly, hips and thighs. Rotate sites each time to ensure optimal transmission of hormones through the skin.

  - If you apply it with your hands, wash your hands thoroughly afterwards to prevent "sharing."

- If you are sleeping with a partner or child, or anticipate skin contact, be sure to apply the hormone at a time when you can cover the area or leave it for at least 4 hours. Then wash the application area before exposing the area to contact with others or before going to bed.

HORMONE CYCLING

Although certain brand name hormone products recommend using a steady low dose, your doctor may suggest you mimic the normal fluctuations of estrogen and progesterone using the bio-identical supplements or prescriptions.

CYCLE METHODS

One method of cycling follows the typical 28 day pattern and it requires the use of oral or cream products. During the first two weeks you will ramp up on estrogen to a peak on day 14 that corresponds to the day ovulation would have taken place. Then you may bring you estrogen dosing down somewhat as you begin ramping up on progesterone for the nest two weeks. At the end of the 4th week, you will reduce both estrogen and progesterone. If you still have a uterus, you should get a period at that time.

I use a modified cycle that runs for two weeks instead of four and which allows me to use the bio-identical estrogen patch (Vivelle Dot) that I find so convenient, plus an OTC progesterone cream. I am currently in the process of testing and documenting this regimen and will report the results on my website (www.HormoneGuru.com) when they are available.

ESTROGEN SURGE NEEDED FOR PROGESTERONE AND TESTOSTERONE

Both types of cycles provide one key benefit that a steady low dose of hormones cannot: they produce an estrogen surge similar to the one that occurs naturally at ovulation. This surge makes it easier for your cells to use both progesterone and testosterone. Without this surge your progesterone and testosterone may be unable to get into your cells where they can do their jobs.

HERBALS AND FOODS

Many solutions have been suggested for relief of the classic symptoms of menopause. But since those are caused by estrogen deficiency or withdrawal, the only fully effective solution is estrogen supplementation.

However, a few substances can help take the edge off these symptoms.

- **Black cohosh.** This is one of the few symptom-relieving herbal solutions that does not contain plant estrogens.

- **Soy and soy products.** Soy contains phytoestrogens which offer mild estrogenic effects. Be aware that some soy products are so overprocessed that their estrogens are lost.

- **Red clover.** This also contains a variety of components that operate like weak estrogens.

WHAT YOU NEED TO KNOW

- Over the counter "progesterone" creams *must* contain *USP progesterone* in order to deliver the benefits of bio-identical progesterone to your body. Although USP progesterone is made from a certain kind of yam, you cannot get progesterone into your system by consuming yams or using products that have only yams in them.

- Though fairly weak, plant estrogens carry the same risks as any other estrogens and they need to be balanced by a sufficiently high level of progesterone (E:P ratio of between 1:35 and 1:75).

- Be aware that you may ingest a number of estrogenic substances from foods (plant estrogens and hormones injected in meat animals) and from manmade plastics (especially when you microwave foods in them or drink water from them). Again, the more estrogens you consume, the more you need progesterone to offset them.

- While lab tests will reflect the levels of human and bio-*identical* hormones in your system, they cannot reflect any bio-*deviant* hormones, including plant estrogens, horse estrogens or plastic estrogens. So be sure you are getting enough progesterone to offset all these hidden substances that mimic estrogen.

Sleep Solutions

One of the most frustrating challenges you may face on a nightly basis is insomnia or poor quality sleep. As you get older, the problem increases as you wake in the night to cool off from a nocturnal heat wave, or to make a trip to the bathroom.

The first step is, obviously, to resolve the causes of those disruptions. But when you've done all you can, or cannot directly address the disruptions, there are a few techniques that can deliver the holy grail of a good night's sleep.

HORMONES

- **Estrogen (estradiol/E2)** is the gold standard for restoring sleep in those having menopausal sleep problems.
- **Melatonin** is nature's original sleeping potion.
- **Progesterone**, especially when taken in oral form at bedtime, can cause drowsiness to help you get to sleep.

OTC DRUGS

Many women resort to taking over-the-counter sleep medicines, and too often they end up taking drugs they don't need that can damage their bodies over time.

WHAT YOU NEED TO KNOW

- OTC sleep aids may be okay to use occasionally, but in the long run they can interfere with your normal sleep processes.

- Nearly all OTC sleep products use antihistamines to induce drowsiness. The most common of these are:
  - Diphenhydramine (Benadryl)
  - Dimenhydrinate (Dramamine)
  - Cetirizine (Zyrtec)
  - Doxylamine (Unisom)

- Many of the sleep aids, like Tylenol PM, contain pain relievers (NSAIDS) as well as an antihistamine like diphenhydramine. These *NSAIDS* are well known to *cause liver damage* when they are used either in high doses for a short time or in low doses over a long period. So please *do not take* a combo like this unless you really need the pain relief. Find out what the sleep ingredient is and get a product that contains *only* that ingredient (or simply switch to melatonin).

HERBS AND AMINO ACIDS

- **Tryptophan.** L-tryptophan is an amino acid in certain protein foods (like turkey) and supplements that can break down into the neurotransmitter serotonin, which in turn breaks down into melatonin. It's best to take tryptophan supplements with no more than a light snack (no protein) and water.

- **Valerian**. Some may recommend valerian for sleep problems, but while it can be effective in causing initial drowsiness, valerian has not been shown effective for overall sleep improvement.

LIFESTYLE

Several changes in your environment and behavior can help promote restful sleep.

SLOW EXERCISE

Though it may sound counterintuitive, for those who lead stressful lives, one of the best things you can do to promote sleep is exercise in the evening before bed.

The key is to perform a slow, steady, non-stimulating exercise — walking on a treadmill for about 30-60 minutes, or bouncing gently on a mini-trampoline for 10-20 minutes shortly before bed. This helps your body burn off any leftover adrenalin, which would otherwise keep you awake.

Just be sure to keep your heart rate *under* 100 beats per minute.

SLEEP HYGIENE

You may hear the term "sleep hygiene" and wonder what it means. Well it's not about washing your armpits or brushing your teeth. In this case, *hygiene* refers to the conditions under which you expect to sleep and how changing those conditions can improve the quantity and quality of your sleep.

- Go to bed at the same time every night.
- Avoid caffeine, tea, chocolate and other stimulants after 5 pm (or earlier, if you are sensitive).
- Avoid stimulating subjects (discussions/arguments, paying bills, TV shows) near bedtime.
- Read or listen to something soothing.
- Take a bath or shower or do something that is calming.

ENVIRONMENT

The pineal gland in your body senses light and determines which hormones to produce based on the light levels around you. So you can help it do its job by controlling the lights you are exposed to in the evening.

Remember that the artificial lighting in your environment tricks your body into thinking it is still daylight even after the sun goes down. So to help simulate a more natural light/dark cycle, here are a few things you can do:

- **Dim the lights after dinner.** Tell your body that the sun is going down. It will start to shift gears gently and will slowly begin to make melatonin, just as if you lived only by the cycles of the sun.

  - If you watch TV in the evening, turn off your room lighting and let the TV provide the primary light.

  - Keep a nightlight in your bathroom so you can brush your teeth and take care of business in the evening without turning on a bright light. You may also want to keep one in the kitchen if you are a midnight snacker.

- **Avoid bluish and green lights in the evening.** The pineal gland is primarily sensitive to blue (and certain green) wavelengths of light (because daylight is in the blue range). So it's best to reduce your exposure to bluish lights in the evening.

  - If you use fluorescent lights indoors, try using bulbs that are warmer (redder) in color rather than the daylight-emulating (bluish) bulbs, at least in your living room, bathroom and other rooms where you spend the most time prior to sleep.

  - If you have nightlights, avoid those that project blue or green colors. Use pink bulbs or red lights instead.

- If you need a clock with a lighted display, get one that displays in red, rather than blue or green.

- Turn off the TV when you go to sleep. TV light overall leans toward the blue wavelengths. So having the TV on tells your brain that it's daylight all night long and to continue producing cortisol to keep you alert. Turning the TV off tells your brain to make relaxing melatonin.

- **Completely darken your bedroom.** If the pineal gland in the brain senses any light, it will slow melatonin production and will order the adrenals to produce cortisol, which can wake you up or prevent you from reaching the most restorative levels of sleep. When you need a really good night's sleep, completely darken your bedroom. Cover up clock displays, power lights, block out street lights, and turn off nightlights.

Urinary Tract Solutions

Urinary tract infections (UTIs) can cause several disturbing symptoms including:

- Constant pressure to urinate, even when your bladder is empty
- Burning/painful urination
- Abdominal pain

UTIs are typically caused when bacteria get into the bladder or urinary tract. The most common invaders are bacteria from the gut (like normal E-coli) that are introduced to the genital area through feces. Those bacteria can be transferred to the urethra either by wiping, through the movement of tight clothing, or (most commonly) by sexual activity.

PREVENTION

The best way to deal with UTIs is to avoid getting them in the first place. And there are a few great ways to help achieve that:

- **Clean thoroughly after bowel movements.** You may have been told to wipe front to back after a BM. This may be all you need. But if you have recurrent UTIs, you may want to use moist towelettes (or even install a bidet) to ensure you remove all bowel bacteria after using the bathroom.

- **Avoid thongs**, jeans and other tight clothing that could transfer fecal bacteria into vaginal and urethral openings as you walk, sit or exercise.

- **Drink cranberry juice** or take cranberry extract to help alter the pH balance of your urinary tract.

- **Wash before sex.** (Doctors refer to UTIs caused by frequent intercourse as "honeymoon cystitis.") Yes, having to stop and wash your (and your partner's) genitals before lovemaking can dampen the mood. But having frequent UTIs will kill the mood for sure. Some women who routinely get UTIs after sex may actually become afraid of sex. So it is well worth the extra time. And if you are creative, you and your partner can find fun, sexy ways to make the washing part of the foreplay.

- **Drink water and urinate before and after sex.** Drinking an 8 oz glass of water before sex puts fluid into your system that will help you flush out any invading bacteria afterwards. Be sure to urinate before having sex to flush out any bacteria that might have started the climb into your pipes. And then urinate again shortly after sex. You don't have to jump out of bed right away, but be sure to potty before going to sleep or getting dressed.

TREATMENT

Once you have a UTI, the whole world may come to a stop until you have found relief from the symptoms. But you also need to treat the cause. Your doctor will typically prescribe antibiotics for a stubborn UTI, but you may be able to resolve the problem on your own using these complementary solutions:

- **Drink lots of water.** It may seem counterintuitive to drink water when you already feel as if you have to pee all the time. But it can feel worse to potty when you have nothing to release. Water also helps dilute the bacteria and flushes your system.

- **Take Azo/phenazopyridine.** The first thing to do while waiting for antibacterial solutions to kick in is to take a product like Azo that numbs your urinary tract (and turns your pee orange). Azo is available at most drug stores. Just follow directions on the package.

- **D-mannose.** Normally the E. coli bacteria latch onto the wall of the bladder and feed on sugars it finds there. But when you take D-mannose (a special type of sugar that bacteria love), the bacteria let go of the small supplies in the bladder and greedily jump into the river of sugar flowing through your urine, riding it like a water slide all way out of your body. D-mannose can be found at most health foods stores. Take 3 to 5 grams (3000-5000 mg) with plenty of water every 3-4 hours while you are awake until the symptoms are gone. If you still have symptoms after about 24 hours, you may need to see a doctor.

Weight Management

For some of us, weight has always been a problem. But as we age, even the skinniest among us begin to face weight problems we'd never dealt with before.

Although it is outside the scope of this book to go into great detail about weight management, a few key solutions are worth mentioning here.

HORMONES

Everything seems to start with hormones. And this subject is no exception. The hormone deficiencies and imbalances in our bodies as we get older make it even harder to keep our bodies in shape. The key hormone solutions that can help are:

- **Increase progesterone, testosterone, DHEA.** These hormones are anabolic, meaning they build lean muscle, which takes up less space in your body and burns fat more efficiently. They also help curb your appetite, especially testosterone. DHEA may also provide some of these benefits because it breaks down into testosterone.

- **Balance estrogen**. Estrogen, by itself, encourages your body to store fat and weaken muscles. So although you need estrogen, you also need testosterone and a lot more progesterone to offset those estrogen effects.

SUPPLEMENTS

There are only a few supplements that may help you safely manage your weight.

CHROMIUM

Chromium is an essential trace mineral that affects insulin and helps regulate blood sugar. Chromium can suppress your cravings for sugar and other simple carbs.

- Take 5000-6000 mcg a day until your cravings subside, then reduce dosage to 1000 mcg/day for maintenance.

ACETYL-L-CARNITINE

Acetyl-l-carnitine (ALC) supports memory and improves stress tolerance. But most important here: it promotes the metabolism of fat, encouraging your body to burn fat, instead of carbs, for fuel.

ALC optimizes insulin so that blood sugar (glucose) can be more effectively metabolized, even in type 2 diabetics.

ALC has been shown to rejuvenate your primary metabolic organ—the liver—which helps you metabolize calories the way you did when you were younger.

OTHERS

- **Relora**. Although products containing Relora tout their ability to reduce belly fat by reducing cortisol, their impact on weight loss has been somewhat disappointing. It may, however offer some appetite-reducing and calming benefits.

- **Sprinkles**. If you are tempted to try a product that claims you can eat normally and lose weight by sprinkling a magic substance on your food, save your money. Although the research the ads talk about is real, the product being advertised does not contain the substances ("tastants") that were actually used in the research! Furthermore, some of these *tastants* that were used in the study are *excitotoxins*, like MSG, that can kill brain cells.

LIFESTYLE

If you are concerned with your weight, you already know that you have to balance calorie intake with exercise. The more you exercise, the more you can consume without gaining weight.

Here are a few more tips:

- As a rule of thumb, it takes about 10 calories to maintain each pound you carry. So to maintain 120 pounds, you must consume at least 1200 calories (depending upon how much exercise you get and how well your metabolism works). Likewise, if you consume 2000 calories a day and don't exercise, you will probably level out at around 200 pounds.

- To keep your metabolism steadily burning calories, especially from fat, eat small meals approximately every 3 hours (5-6 small meals daily), ideally with a little protein in each, heavy on fresh fruits and vegetables, with some nuts and whole grains.

- If you know you will be indulging in a meal high in simple carbs (sugar, bread, pasta, etc.), take a dose of a fiber supplement (e.g., psyllium) before the meal to fill you up and help keep your blood sugar levels steady.

WHAT YOU NEED TO KNOW

- **Low-carb diets**. Be careful with low-carb, high-protein diets. Protein metabolizes into acids which can change the pH of your blood, which causes your body to pull calcium out of bones and muscles to neutralize the acid. Bottom line: high protein diets can weaken bones (and cause kidney stones) over time. It's okay to use them for a few weeks to kick-start your weight loss, but be sure to transition into a healthier, more balanced diet after that.

- **Fat doesn't make you fat**. Your body needs healthy fats for any number of critical functions. And reducing the fat in your diet cannot help you lose weight. It is all about calories *consumed* versus calories *burned*.

- **Carbs in moderation.** Carbohydrates are easier for your body to burn, so when you feed it carbs (especially sugar and flour), you make your metabolism lazy and keep it from having to work harder to burn fat stores. It's like building a campfire with nothing but dry leaves. You will have to keep feeding the fire more and more leaves and it will never be able to get the longer-lasting logs burning. Reducing or eliminating simple carbs from your diet can yield dramatic results both in terms of cravings and weight reduction.

- **Eat like a diabetic**. Possibly the healthiest solution ever for losing and maintaining your weight is the diabetic diet. Diabetics help manage their blood sugar by eating several small meals and snacks throughout the day—meals that are low in refined sugar and flour and that include protein and lots of fresh fruits and vegetables.

Bottom Line

Share these secrets with your healthcare team and make sure they understand and support your goals.

There's no time like the present to start feeling like the phenomenal woman you are!

Contact

Please feel free to contact me and share your experiences at: **www. HormoneGuru.com**.

I look forward to hearing from you!

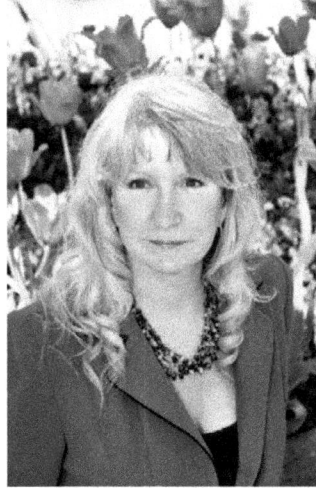

Patricia Copley O'Connell is a professional writer with a gift for making complex subjects easy to understand. Her previous book for medical professionals detailed cutting-edge advances in anti-aging and hormone therapy. Now she makes these insider secrets accessible to every woman over 35 who wants to stay young, healthy and vibrant.

www. HormoneGuru.com

www.ingramcontent.com/pod-product-compliance
Lightning Source LLC
Chambersburg PA
CBHW072118270326
41931CB00010B/1595